SUPERFOOD
NUTS

SUPERFOOD
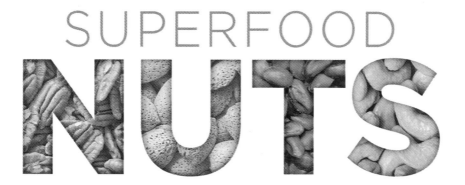
NUTS

A Guide to Cooking with Power-Packed Walnuts, Almonds, Pecans, and More

Connie Diekman
MEd, RD, CSSD, LD, FAND

Vicki Chelf

Foreword by
Daniel Rosenberg, PhD

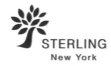

STERLING
New York

STERLING
New York

An Imprint of Sterling Publishing, Co., Inc.
1166 Avenue of the Americas
New York, NY 10016

ISBN 978-1-4549-2334-3

Distributed in Canada by Sterling Publishing Co., Inc.
c/o Canadian Manda Group, 664 Annette Street
Toronto, Ontario, Canada M6S 2C8
Distributed in the United Kingdom by GMC Distribution Services
Castle Place, 166 High Street, Lewes, East Sussex, England BN7 1XU
Distributed in Australia by NewSouth Books
45 Beach Street, Coogee, NSW 2034, Australia

For information about custom editions, special sales, and premium and corporate purchases,
please contact Sterling Special Sales at 800-805-5489 or specialsales@sterlingpublishing.com.

Manufactured in Canada

2 4 6 8 10 9 7 5 3 1

www.sterlingpublishing.com

CONTENTS

FOREWORD

As the director of Colon Cancer Prevention at UConn Health, I oversee a program that offers patients entry into a clinical study of early-stage abnormal growths in the colon, among other things. Patients who consent to the study fill out a questionnaire that asks for a breakdown of their tree nut consumption. Patients also provide a blood specimen and answer a series of demographic questions about their overall health and risk factors for colon cancer, such as their BMI, waist-to-hip ratio, smoking history, and NSAID intake. The patient is then provided with a state-of-the-art colonoscopy examination using a high-definition endoscope and contrast dye-spray to illuminate the bowel wall and provide images of even microscopic lesions. We remove up to ten of these lesions and then study their biology in the laboratory. We also have a number of mouse genetic models of colon cancer that we routinely use in the laboratory to gain a better understanding of the earliest stages of GI cancer. Using the models, we have defined a number of nutritional variables that may contribute to cancer risk, including the levels of folic acid.

Our interest in exploring novel ways to reduce cancer risk in people began several decades ago when the relatively new field of cancer prevention with the use of natural products and non-toxic synthetic agents (e.g., aspirin) was in its earliest days. In the 1960s the field of cancer "prophylaxis" was created by the insights of Dr. Lee Wattenberg. It was later refined in the 1970s by Dr. Michael B. Sporn, who coined the term cancer "chemoprevention" while working at the National Cancer Institute. Spurred by the realization that a wide variety of natural products could have a beneficial effect on a person's risk for developing myriad cancers, we launched our research program to find new mechanisms that could be exploited for cancer prevention. Progress in this field of research over the past few decades has been extraordinary, with many new approaches developed that may ultimately contribute to the eradication of cancer.

One such strategy that has been under intense scrutiny in recent years is the health benefit of consuming what we generally refer to as the Mediterranean Diet, a way of eating that is rich in fruits and vegetables, legumes, fish, and olive oil (Fazio and Ricciardiello, *Phytochemistry Reviews*, 2014). One key ingredient of the Mediterranean Diet is the tree nut. Of the various tree nuts, walnuts offer a remarkably healthy nutritional composition, including ellagitannins, vitamin E, omega-3 fatty acids, polyphenols, phytosterols, melatonin, and fiber. We have recently tested the potential for walnuts to protect against intestinal cancer using a mouse genetic model in our laboratory (Nakanishi et al., *Cancer Prevention Research*, 2016). We reported that walnuts added to a "Western style" diet loaded with a number of common fats found in the American diet and less calcium and vitamins provided protection against cancer development. Not only that, but the walnuts actually acted like a "probiotic" agent, causing a remarkable change to the community structure of the intestinal microbiota. We are excited by these recent findings and have initiated a series of related studies to test the beneficial effects of walnuts in a second mouse cancer model, as well as an experimental model of inflammatory bowel disease.

I believe this book is extremely timely and of great importance to the general population. Offering a natural and healthy way to potentially reduce risk of cancer by simply incorporating an outstanding nutritional source (that is, tree nuts) into your diet makes sense, both from the nutritional standpoint and from a scientific perspective.

—Daniel W. Rosenberg, PhD
Professor of Medicine and Health Net, Inc.
Chair in Cancer Biology
Investigator, Center for Molecular Medicine
University of Connecticut School of Medicine

As you read the title of this book, you might think, "How can nuts be super when you consider the fat that they contain or the salt that is on them?" Nuts were lauded as a key component of the diet, then feared for their fat, and have now regained favor as an element of healthy eating.

Nuts are a versatile food. You can eat them by themselves, include them in recipes, or feature them as an accent to dishes. Nuts offer a wide variety of nutrients, including protein, which makes them good additions to any eating plan. But there are two things that make them "superfoods": fats and phytonutrients.

Nuts are composed of a variety of fats; and while each nut variety has a different fat composition, they all tend to have more of the healthier, unsaturated fats. Unsaturated fats are found predominantly in plants: vegetable oils, nuts, and seeds. Unsaturated fats are liquid at room temperature; so if you were to take the fat out of a nut, it would be liquid at room temperature. Research shows that unsaturated fats provide more heart health benefits than saturated fats, including helping to lower blood cholesterol, fighting inflammation, helping with heart rhythm, and other health-promoting benefits.

All nuts contain unsaturated fat, but some have more than others. Some nuts have more of the less healthful saturated fats, and in subsequent chapters we will talk more about these differences among the nuts. Saturated fats are solid at room temperature, and consuming too much of them has been associated with an increased risk of heart disease. The ideal way to include nuts in your eating plan is to learn which ones provide more of the unsaturated fat and simply use those nuts more often. These are what I call "Superfood Nuts." As you read through this book you will see that there is more evidence of the health benefits of certain nuts. This might simply be the fact that some nuts are more healthful than others, but it could also point to the types of nuts researchers choose to study or the availability of nuts for researchers to do strong enough and large enough studies.

Besides being rich in unsaturated fats, Superfood Nuts are composed of beneficial phytonutrients. Phytonutrients are plant compounds that provide health benefits beyond those provided by the vitamins and minerals contained in the food. Over the last several years research studies have looked at plant foods to try to understand why they provide so many health benefits that exceed their basic nutrition profile. Though all the answers aren't in yet, research shows that phytonutrients, which make each plant food unique, are used in many different ways by the body to fight inflammation, help prevent disease, aid intestinal health, and even help with memory, among other things.

In *Superfood Nuts*, we have tried to make nutrition facts simple. So while we will look at the nutrient profile of nuts, the discussion will focus on the complete potential health benefits package that each nut provides. In addition, we will outline which nuts are healthier choices based on the evidence of their role in health promotion. The recipes demonstrate how you can make nuts a part of your everyday meal plan, not just a snack here or there. Talking about and sharing the science of good nutrition and nuts are important aspects of what I do as a registered dietitian, and it is also a part of the passion I have. Telling you that nuts are good for you is one thing, but helping you understand the science behind that statement can make it easier for you to understand how nuts fit into a healthful eating plan. Few people think about science when they make food choices, but I hope the information in this book will help you think about the amount and variety of plant foods you eat, the diversity of nuts in your diet, and how to find balance between your overall nutrient intake and the calories that you allocate to nuts.

A fun aspect of writing this book was the chance to talk about nutrition and develop recipes with a very nice—and talented—chef. Chef Vicki not only has a passion for creating delectable recipes but she understands the importance of good nutrition (not the latest nutrition fad), values the science behind it, and likes to develop recipes that convey her passion, talent, and knowledge. Here in her words Chef Vicki shares her excitement about creating the recipes in this book.

In the kitchen, nuts are magic! From the savory and crunchy to the sweet and creamy, nuts can expand your menu to include healthy and delicious dishes in ways that you may not have considered, as the fat in nuts can take the place of extracted oils in many recipes. Imagine thin, crispy whole-grain crackers, creamy soups and sauces without milk, cream, or butter, and robust salad dressings all made from blended nuts. Nuts also add a satisfying and meaty quality to main dishes, yet they are totally plant-based and vegetarian.

Almond milk is popular, and making it yourself, with the easy instructions in this book, saves money and allows you to use the whole nut. The leftover pulp can be made into a delicious spread or garnish that I call Faux Chèvre Frais (page 43).

In *Superfood Nuts* you will find loads of other recipes for more conventional ways to use nuts in baked goods, toppings, and desserts. These recipes are special because they contain whole grain, rather than refined flour, and are lower in fat and sugar than what is typical. The baked goods in this book are also made without dairy products or eggs, so people with allergies, as well as vegans, may enjoy them. Many of the breads and almost all the desserts are gluten-free, too.

The recipes in this book have been a joy to create. Nuts are so delicious to begin with that adding them to all sorts of dishes simply enhances the recipe. These recipes are easy and quick to make, because I am busy and I know that you are, too. I do hope that you find the time to try each and every one of them. Then, like me, you can go super nuts over *Superfood Nuts*!

As you can see through her words, Chef Vicki loves creating and experimenting with foods to develop recipes that offer different options but plenty of nutrition. Her passion for creativity and my passion for the science of nutrition have come together nicely to provide you with information about nut nutrition and to help you enjoy some new, healthful recipes that reflect the science behind the benefits of nuts.

What better way to wrap up our introduction than to say that we both hope you find our words and recipes an inspiration, a base of knowledge, and an excellent starting point to get some Super Taste, Super Nutrition, and Super Excitement about nuts. Bon Appetit!

—Connie Diekman,
M.Ed., RD, CSSD, LD, FADA,
nutrition communications consultant

—Vicki Chelf,
author and chef

CHAPTER 1

HEALTH BENEFITS OF NUTS

Nuts, as a category, are nutrient-rich foods, making them good choices in any diet. But in addition to their rich nutrient package they contain a wide variety of phytonutrients, which further enhance the role they can play in maintenance of health and possibly prevention of disease.

As we look at nuts in health, you will see that different nuts provide different health benefits, and some nuts seem to possess more benefits than others. This difference is likely a function of the differences in phytonutrients, but it might also be the difference in the amount of research conducted with different nuts. In looking at health benefits, we will discuss the unique nutrient package of most tree nuts and provide an overview of the health benefits that are unique to each. Overall studies of nuts and their health benefits have generally examined their role in these six categories: some types of cancer, cardiovascular disease, cognitive function, diabetes, diet quality, and weight.

HEALTH TIP: Phytonutrients are many in number and are found in all plant foods, which is one of the reasons that the 2015 *Dietary Guidelines for Americans* by the US Department of Health and Human Services recommends consuming half your plate from fruits and vegetables and a bit more than a quarter of your plate from grains, with half of those grains coming from whole grains. In addition, the guidelines suggest choosing unsalted nuts and seeds as a part of a healthier eating plan.

Nut phytonutrients will not change an otherwise poor eating plan, so make sure you add them to an overall healthful eating plan, don't just expect them to work magic.

HEALTH TIP: When deciding which nuts to include in your eating plan, consider tree nuts, which provide a wide variety of benefits. Tree nuts include almonds, Brazil nuts, cashews, hazelnuts, macadamias, pecans, pine nuts, pistachios, and walnuts. Peanuts are actually legumes; while they offer many health benefits, they are not included here because this book focuses only on tree nuts.

CANCER

Several studies have looked at the connection between nut consumption and cancer incidence and mortality. The studies have varied in size, duration, subject demographics, and outcomes. Some of them have been observational, so they are not designed to determine cause and effect but instead provide evidence that is worth looking at further. Outcomes have been mixed: Some of the studies have shown a connection between nut consumption and a lower risk of cancer and death from cancer, while others have not demonstrated any connection. The very large 2015 PREDIMED trial looked at a small sample of only women to see if nut consumption (supplementing a Mediterranean diet) reduced risk of invasive breast cancer, but the outcome was inconclusive.

HEALTH TIP: Research studies vary in design, but one frequently used method is the observational study. Observational studies are not designed to determine if something caused an outcome to happen but are simply designed to give researchers insight into a research question. If an observation indicates a trend, then a further study designed to measure cause and effect would be the next step. Observational studies are often used to broach questions about diet, since they help determine whether dietary changes affect health. However, they do not provide a basis for recommendations. Instead, they provide interesting outcomes that point the way toward more systematic studies.

RANDOMIZED CONTROL TRIALS

When looking at research studies, randomized control trials (RCTs) provide the best study design and are therefore more likely to show a true outcome. RCTs often are expensive to conduct and take a longer period of time to show an outcome, making them less desirable to fund. Other study designs can provide some indications of possible outcomes, but it is important to remember that many studies show trends or indications, not cause and effect, so always check a study design before trusting an outcome. When a media report talks about a new study, do the following:

1. Check to see what type of study it was.

2. Check to see how long the study lasted.

3. Check to see how many people were in the study.

Studies that are small, short-term, and not designed to provide cause-and-effect outcome should be viewed as interesting, not a recommendation for change.

CARDIOVASCULAR DISEASE

Research in the area of cardiovascular disease has been extensive with studies going back more than thirty years. Studies have looked at consumption of most tree nuts but most of the research has been done with almonds and walnuts. While study designs have varied from long-term, randomized trials to short-term, nonrandomized trials, outcomes tend to show the same thing: Those who consume nuts tend to have a lower incidence of heart disease and stroke, have better blood lipid levels, and have a lower death rate caused by cardiovascular disease.

In 2013 Harvard medical school published results of a study in more than 70,000 female nurses and more than 42,000 men in the Health Professionals Follow-up Study in which nut consumption was associated with a reduction in total deaths and disease-specific deaths. The study found that those who consumed one ounce of nuts seven or more times a week had a 20 percent lower death rate than those who ate fewer nuts. The study also found that those who consumed more nuts were leaner and tended to have a healthier lifestyle than those who consumed fewer nuts. While the study was only observational, with no cause-and-effect outcome, the fact that there was a connection between nut consumption and reduced death is an interesting note.

The PREDIMED trial is the most recent large-scale study demonstrating that consumption of nuts—walnuts, hazelnuts, and almonds—was associated with a decreased risk of death from cardiovascular disease. PREDIMED studied nut consumption by more than 7,000 men and women for an average of almost five years and measured the number of cardiovascular events during that time. The study found that subjects who consumed the nuts, specifically walnuts, hazelnuts, and almonds, had fewer cardiovascular events, suggesting a benefit from the nuts.

In 2015 a multi-university study compiled the outcomes of three large cohort studies to determine the impact of nut consumption on total number of deaths as well as cause of death. The three studies included the Southern Community Cohort Study of more than 70,000 southeastern US residents of African and European descent, who were predominately lower economic class residents, the Shanghai Women's Health Study, and the Shanghai Men's Health Study; the Shanghai studies totaled more than 130,000 participants. The average length of follow-up was just over six years. Outcomes from the complied data showed an overall decrease in cardiovascular disease deaths among all groups who consumed nuts.

HEALTH TIP: A heart-healthy diet is more than just adding nuts to an eating plan. It is a diet that includes more plant foods— whole grains, fruits, and vegetables *and* for the protein choices: either leaner, lower-fat animal foods or plant-based proteins like beans, nuts, seeds, and soy. Choosing to enjoy a plant-based diet or to include animal foods can meet nutrient needs; it is a matter of balance. In addition, healthy body weight and regular physical activity are also key parts of a lifestyle that reduces the risk of heart disease. No one food will provide health magic, so if you are adding nuts to reduce risk of heart disease, make sure your overall diet is heart healthy.

LABEL CLAIMS ON NUTS

In 2003 the Food and Drug Administration reviewed the body of scientific evidence related to nuts and cardiovascular disease and ruled that "Scientific evidence suggests but does not prove that eating 1.5 ounces per day of most nuts [such as *name of specific nut*] as part of a diet low in saturated fat and cholesterol may reduce the risk of heart disease. [See nutrition information for fat content.]" This claim can appear on packages of nuts or any materials associated with the promotion or sale of nuts. Learn more about label claims in the Resources section.

HEALTH TIP: In the 2015 *Dietary Guidelines for Americans*, the evolving evidence on fat and its role in heart disease risk is reflected by the removal of an upper limit for daily fat consumption in terms of percent of calories from fat. While this is a good change, what is important is that the type of fats you choose should be unsaturated, found predominantly in plant foods. Nuts, along with seeds and nut oils, provide healthier fat choices than animal fats.

The 2015 *Guidelines* might not suggest a limit to the amount of fat you eat, it does provide the reminder that consuming too much fat has an impact on calorie intake, which can affect weight and ultimately, overall health.

COGNITIVE FUNCTION

As baby boomers age, research is evolving on the possible role of nuts in preventing memory loss and preserving cognitive function. Alzheimer's is the fifth leading cause of death in Americans age 65 and older and incidence is expected to grow. While there is currently no clear way to prevent Alzheimer's or dementia, research has begun to look at ways that diet might delay the onset of disease and maintain mental acuity. A few studies have reported observations on nuts and mental health and a few more are in progress.

Studies that have been completed show a connection between nut consumption and preserved cognition. One study looked at close to 450 adults, ages 55 to 80, and found that those who consumed walnuts, but no other types of nuts, had a better working memory. Researchers theorized that the phytonutrient content of walnuts is the reason they showed a positive benefit. But the study was observational in design, so more research is needed to determine cause and effect.

Researchers at Tufts University also looked at walnuts and mental function. While the study yielded a positive outcome, it was small in size. Larger studies of longer duration are needed.

HEALTH TIP

For reputable health professionals to make a recommendation about a food and/or a health recommendation, scientific evidence must be significant. A significant body of evidence exists when many studies have shown the same outcome. The quality of the studies is also important. For evidence to be conclusive, studies should be done in a variety of populations, in males and females, in different age groups, and should be designed to yield a clear outcome. These factors are some of the reasons that making claims about food and health take so long. If you don't want to try to figure out if a study is a good scientific recommendation, contact a registered dietitian for help with food and nutrition information.

DIABETES

Diabetes continues to be a major health problem. One key way to control and/or prevent diabetes is to make dietary changes. Studies have looked at whether consumption of nuts can reduce the incidence of diabetes. Though it did not focus on nut consumption alone, the PREDIMED trial is the most recent study to provide a small-scale look at nut consumption and blood sugar levels. The PREDIMED trial found that consuming extra-virgin olive oil or eating walnuts, hazelnuts, and almonds on a daily basis both helped lower blood sugar levels and boosted control of diabetes, but there was no clear benefit from nuts alone. Other trials have looked at nut consumption and risk of death due to diabetes and have found no clear connection.

A large-scale study from Harvard University in 2013 found that regular consumption of nuts, particularly walnuts, as a part of a healthy diet, is associated with a lower incidence of type 2 diabetes. The study followed close to 60,000 older women and close to 80,000 younger women who were free of diabetes at the start of the study. The study followed the women for ten years with assessments of food intake every four years during the study.

The outcome of the study showed a reduction in risk of development of type 2 diabetes in the women who consumed nuts more often. This study, like several of the others, was observational in design, so declaring a cause-and-effect outcome was not possible, but the indication that nut consumption lowered the risk of type 2 diabetes is important.

HEALTH TIP: One of the main causes of type 2 diabetes is being overweight, so until more evidence demonstrates a cause-and-effect outcome between nuts and prevention, focus on achieving and maintaining a healthy body weight. Achieving a healthy body weight is best accomplished by following an eating plan that is flexible, enjoyable, and one that meets your nutrient needs. In addition, regular physical activity is a key part of keeping weight within a normal range, so make sure you find a type of activity that fits your lifestyle and that your physician says is safe for you to do.

HEALTH TIP: Type 2 diabetes used to be referred to as a disease of middle age, but as more and more Americans are becoming overweight, type 2 diabetes is developing in younger adults. Approximately 10 percent of the US population has type 2 diabetes and 28 percent of the population has undiagnosed type 2 diabetes. Body fat does not allow insulin to move blood glucose into body cells, so the glucose stays in the blood system, leading to blood readings that show high levels of blood sugar. Working to lower body fat and boost muscle mass is a good way to improve insulin function and lower blood sugar. Don't take any chance if you haven't had your blood sugar checked. Instead, take some time to learn about your risk level.

HEALTH TIP: An area of confusion when it comes to diet and diabetes is the inclusion of carbohydrates. Carbohydrates are essential body fuel, but the wrong types of carbohydrates or too much carbohydrate can trigger problems for those with diabetes. While your physician and registered dietitian should guide your meal planning, consuming carbohydrates from whole grains, vegetables, beans, nuts, and seeds should be the first line of defense. Carbohydrates from fruits provide nutritional value, so they are better choices, for instance, than carbohydrates from simple sugars such as candy, table sugar, honey, and sugar-sweetened beverages. In addition, watching portions is important.

HEALTH TIP: Carbohydrates are often referred to as "simple" or "complex." Simple carbohydrates are made up of only two chemical molecules, so they provide a quicker source of fuel. The molecules vary, but the bottom line is that simple carbohydrates end up as either glucose, which is then available for the body to use as fuel, or as fructose, which goes to the liver to be broken down to glucose, triglycerides, and glycogen, a storage form of glucose. Simple carbohydrates are found in fruit, milk, and sugars like honey, white sugar, brown sugar, etc.

Complex carbohydrates are long, long molecules that break down into molecules of glucose. Complex carbohydrates provide a slower source of fuel, helping to keep you fueled longer, and are found in grains, vegetables, beans, nuts, and seeds.

DIET QUALITY

Nuts offer such a wide variety of nutrients, it is not surprising that they would be associated with a diet that offers better overall quality. Conducting research to document this makes it easier to give them a callout for their role in boosting diet quality.

In 2015 a study looked at nut intake using food-intake histories of more than 14,000 men and women who provided information to the National Health and Nutrition Examination Survey during the years 2005 to 2010. The national survey looks at diet trends, nutritional adequacy, and any connections between nutrition and disease. The research study reviewed diet recollections to assess tree nut consumption over a two-day period. Results showed that those who consumed nuts more often had a higher fiber and potassium intake and overall diet quality was higher for the group.

This outcome provides evidence that adding nuts might increase calories but the quality of those calories is better than without the nuts.

HEALTH TIP: It is common for people to focus on calorie intake and forget that the quality of the calories they choose is important to overall health, energy levels, and long-term disease prevention. When deciding how to divide up your calories, think about the nutrients in the food you choose. One good way to do that is to use the MyPlate guide (Choosemyplate.gov). Calories certainly do count as they relate to our weight, but if the calories we choose are missing the nutrients we need, overall health is impacted and a healthy weight is not as helpful.

HEALTH TIP: Diet quality is important to overall health but doesn't mean you can't have some "fun foods" or "treats" every so often. It's about meeting nutrient needs over time, so when assessing your diet, look at a day, a week, or even a month to determine if you are consuming calories that are nutrient rich or just calories. When you have reviewed how your nutrition balances out and if you are meeting your body's needs as outlined in the *Dietary Guidelines*, you can choose up to 10 percent of your calories from added sugars found in many fun or treat foods.

WEIGHT

When I talk with clients about nutrition, one of the first things they bring up is weight— what about all the calories nuts contain? Well, there's good news on two fronts. First, if consumed appropriately, nuts do not appear to contribute to weight gain and they may, in fact, help with weight maintenance. Second, new analysis of nuts has shown that the calories indicated in nutrition databases do not reflect the actual number of calories absorbed. So, in actuality, nuts contribute fewer calories than databases state.

Research studies have begun to assess how nuts in the diet might impact weight. One study, which was a collaborative effort of researchers at three universities, looked at weight-loss routines that included nuts and outcomes of those regimens. This observational study found that diets that included nuts improved patient compliance and led to higher weight loss. The researchers theorized that, in addition to aiding weight loss, the increased palatability of nuts might be a reason that people found it easier to adhere to a diet routine.

Several other, smaller studies have shown that inclusion of nuts in the diet does not contribute to weight gain when they are consumed as a part of a healthful, well-balanced diet. The Adventist Health Study found that consuming a one-ounce serving of tree nuts each week was associated with a 7 percent reduction in the occurrence of metabolic syndrome, a condition often triggered by weight gain. This study also found, similar to the Harvard study, that those who consumed more tree nuts had a lower prevalence of obesity.

When it comes to the actual number of calories absorbed from nuts, over the last several years the USDA has conducted studies on nut consumption and caloric absorption for almonds, pistachios, and walnuts. The studies found that almonds and walnuts have about 20 percent fewer absorbed calories than the number of calories listed in nutrient databases and pistachios have about 5 percent fewer calories. While the reason(s) for this is still not clear, USDA researchers theorized that it could be a function of inadequate chewing, making it more difficult to absorb the calories, or it could be due to the fiber content of the nuts.

HOW DO YOU CHEW?

One of the key components of satiety—how full and how satisfied you feel after eating—is how well you chew the foods you eat. Evidence shows that chewing more slowly, pacing the bites you take, and focusing on how food tastes improves your feelings of satisfaction and can help you with weight control. When you enjoy your next meal, take time to look at how the food fills your plate, smell the food, and notice the specialness of the meal. Also notice the texture, colors, and differences of foods on your plate before you start eating.

OTHER POTENTIAL HEALTH BENEFITS

Studies looking at other health benefits of nuts are growing. In addition, researchers are looking at nuts as part of an eating plan that helps older adults maintain physical function, mobility, balance, and more.

Studies have looked at walnut consumption and male fertility where men with fertility issues consumed walnuts for twelve weeks. Outcomes showed improved sperm vitality and motility in the group of men who consumed the walnuts.

The health of our gut is another area of research, with studies looking at the overall health of the gut when nuts are consumed, the impact of nut consumption on development of bowel disorders such as inflammatory bowel disease, and the role of nuts in reducing development of tumors in the gut. Studies in this area are in the very early stages, so many are done using animals, but they're showing exciting outcomes related to gut health. Researchers are pointing to the fiber in nuts, along with the divergent phytonutrient content of nuts, as possible links to a healthier gut environment and subsequent disease prevention. Stay tuned!

HEALTH TIP: The role of nuts in health promotion and disease prevention is still not totally clear, but we know that an eating plan that includes more plant foods is more healthful. While we may not know which nuts do what or how much you should eat or if those nuts will help you, choosing nuts over chips or candy will provide health benefits. No matter how "super" nuts are, their benefit is only as good as how healthful your overall lifestyle is. Don't assume that one change to your diet or the addition of super foods will offset a lifestyle that is otherwise not health promoting.

HEALTH TIP: A healthy gut allows you to feel good and digest foods well, but it also helps strengthen your immune system. A major part—some estimates indicate it could be 70 to 80 percent—of the immune system is located in your gut. While research is still looking at how the gut impacts overall health, it does appear that a diet rich in plant foods—grains, fruits, vegetables, beans, nuts, and seeds—helps promote gut health, which may be another reason that nuts are good for overall health.

HEALTH BENEFITS OF INDIVIDUAL TREE NUTS

We looked at how nuts appear to contribute to overall health, but each nut has a different nutrient profile and impact to overall health. To help you understand how each tree nut is different and what each nut can contribute to your diet, let's walk through the nutrition facts of tree nuts.

ALMONDS

Almonds and pistachios are a bit different from the nuts of other flowering trees in that these nuts develop within a shell that is surrounded by a hull, very much like other stone fruits (also known as drupes). This formation protects the nut.

When it comes to nutrition, almonds provide a wide variety of nutrients, including the major calorie nutrients. According to the US Department of Agriculture, one ounce of almonds, which is about 23 whole nuts, provides the following nutrients.

Calories / 1 ounce serving 163
Protein (g) 6.0
Total Fat (g) 14.0
Saturated Fat (g) 1.1
Monounsaturated Fat (g) 8.8
Polyunsaturated Fat (g) 3.4
Carbohydrates (g) 6.1
Dietary Fiber (g) 3.5
Potassium (mg) 200
Magnesium (mg) 76
Zinc (mg) 0.9
Copper (mg) 0.3
Selenium (mcg) 2.5
Manganese (mg) 0.6
Vitamin B6 (mg) 0
Folate (mcg) 14
Riboflavin (mg) 0.3
Niacin (mg) 1.0
Alpha-tocopherol (mg) 7.4
Calcium (mg) 75
Iron (mg) 1.1

USDA Food Composition Databases. https://ndb.nal.usda.gov/ndb/foods/show/3635?manu=&fgcd=&ds=. Accessed June 26, 2016.

The overall nutrient package of almonds is obvious, but to put the nutrition of almonds in perspective: ounce for ounce, almonds provide the highest amount of protein, fiber, calcium, vitamin E or alpha-tocopherol, riboflavin, and niacin of all nuts, in only 163 calories. In fact, the amount of manganese, magnesium, and vitamin E in almonds is at a level that meets the USDA definition for "excellent source of." According to USDA, for a food to claim "excellent source of" the food must "contain 20 percent or more of the DV (Daily Value)" based on a two-thousand-calorie reference diet. In addition to containing high-level nutrients, the almond is a "good source of" riboflavin, copper, phosphorous, and fiber. The USDA definition for "good source of" is a food

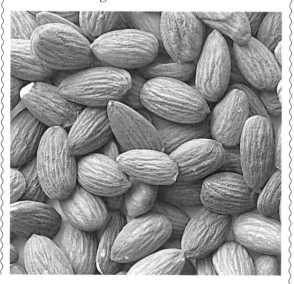

that contain(s) 10 percent to 19 percent of the DV. When you consider that seven of the nutrients in almonds put the nut into such high levels, it is clear why almonds can play a big role in a healthful eating plan.

The fat content of nuts is often an area of concern but what is important is the distribution of that fat into the less healthful saturated fat versus the more healthful unsaturated fat. Almonds provide a limited amount of saturated fat and a high concentration of monounsaturated fats, which likely is the connection between almonds and the reduction in heart disease risk. Monounsaturated fats, along with polyunsaturated fats, can help lower LDL or bad cholesterol levels. Research on the role of almonds and heart disease risk reduction spans more than twenty years with studies of varying size, duration, and intake but conclusions consistently have demonstrated the positive benefit of almonds in reducing LDL levels.

A recent meta-analysis looked at eighteen studies to assess the impact of almonds on blood cholesterol and triglyceride levels. The meta-analysis reported consumption of almonds helped improve blood lipid levels and helped reduce the risk of heart disease. The recent study did not provide a mechanism by which this impact occurred but suggested that the impact might be a result of several factors. The healthful fatty acid profile of almonds might be a reason for the change in blood lipid levels, or it is possible that almond consumption is associated with a healthier body weight

META-ANALYSIS

Meta-analysis is a systematic process that combines the results of similar studies to get an outcome that offers a higher degree of validity. A conclusion from a meta-analysis is statistically of higher significance than a conclusion of a single study. Meta-analysis is the highest level of scientific evidence, and if a meta-analysis includes studies that are randomized control trials (RCTs) the outcome of the meta-analysis would be at the highest level of significance. Meta-analysis of observational studies might provide a more significant outcome than a single observational study—it is still important to remember that observational studies are not designed to yield cause and effect, so the meta-analysis would give an indication, not a cause-and-effect outcome.

or it might be due to the phytonutrient profile of almonds.

As a result of the earlier studies, the Food and Drug Administration (FDA) approved a qualified health claim about the benefit of consuming most nuts and reduction in risk for heart disease. The claim was discussed in the beginning of this chapter but with regard to almonds the specific qualified health claim states, "Scientific evidence suggests, but does not prove, that eating 1.5 ounces per day of most nuts, such as almonds, as part of a diet low in saturated fat and cholesterol may reduce the risk of heart disease." This recent meta-analysis clearly reaffirms the health claim.

BRAZIL NUTS

When we talk about superfood nuts the Brazil nut often is left out of the conversation due to its saturated fat content. The Brazil nut is the large seed of trees that grow in the Amazon jungle. The seed grows in clusters of eight to twenty-four inside a hard shell with a texture (but not a shape) something like a coconut.

The Brazil nut is a high-fat nut and even though it contains about 75 percent unsaturated fat, the healthier type of fat, the remaining saturated fat makes it the highest in saturated fat of any nut. When deciding if you want to consume Brazil nuts, you should focus on how they fit into your eating plan so that the saturated fat that they provide can be offset by other, lower saturated–fat foods.

In terms of nutrients the stars for Brazil nuts are selenium, copper, magnesium, and phosphorus. Their nutrient profile follows. The Brazil nut is an "excellent source of" selenium, actually providing 774 percent of the daily requirement of selenium (the USDA recommends 20 percent). In addition to being an excellent source of copper, magnesium, and phosphorus, it is also a good source of manganese and thiamin.

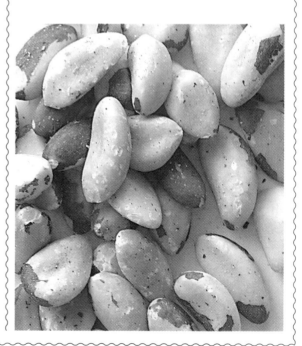

Calories / 1 ounce serving 186
Protein (g) 4.1
Total Fat (g) 18.8
Saturated Fat (g) 4.3
Monounsaturated Fat (g) 7.0
Polyunsaturated Fat (g) 3.5
Carbohydrates (g) 6.1
Dietary Fiber (g) 3.5
Potassium (mg) 187
Magnesium (mg) 107
Zinc (mg) 1.2
Copper (mg) 0.5
Selenium (mcg) 640
Manganese (mg) 0.4
Vitamin B6 (mg) 0
Folate (mcg) 6
Riboflavin (mg) 0
Niacin (mg) 0.1
Alpha-tocopherol (mg) 1.6
Calcium (mg) 45
Iron (mg) 0.7

USDA Food Composition Databases. https://ndb.nal
.usda.gov/ndb/foods/show/3641?manu=&fgcd=&ds=.
Accessed June 26, 2016.

Because selenium is so widely distributed in the food supply, and because the Reference Daily Intake (RDI) is relatively low, deficiencies are uncommon in most Western countries.

Brazil nuts differ from other nuts in that they cannot carry the qualified health claim for nuts. The qualified health claim can only appear on nuts that contain fewer than four grams of saturated fat for a 1.5 ounce or 50 gram serving. Since Brazil nuts contain more than four grams of saturated fat in an ounce they cannot carry the claim.

HEALTH TIP: Due to the high fat content of Brazil nuts, they are very susceptible to rancidity. Prevent rancidity of the Brazil nut, and most nuts, by purchasing only the amount you need, storing them in the refrigerator for up to three months, and storing them in the freezer for up to a year. Be sure to store them in an airtight container to further prevent breakdown of the fat; and remember that each time you open the container, you expose the nuts to air, so the time they stay fresh may diminish. Of many popular nuts, these varieties are most susceptible to rancidity: English walnuts, pecans, Brazil nuts, peanuts, almonds, pistachios, cashews, and hazelnuts.

HEALTH TIP: The mineral selenium, which is found in the soil and water, works with vitamin E to protect cells from damage due to oxidation that can lead to heart disease and some types of cancer. Selenium is in Brazil nuts, meat, seafood, liver, and grains so consuming adequate amounts is generally easy to do. Supplementation should be considered carefully since selenium can be toxic in excess. Ask your physician and/or registered dietitian to determine if you need a supplement.

CASHEWS

Cashews are a bit different from other nuts. Cashews grow as a part of the cashew fruit, which is often referred to as the "cashew apple." The reason for this term is that the cashew fruit truly looks like an apple, though it is more yellow-red in color, and the nut, which is grayish brown in color, hangs from the lower end of the cashew apple. The cashew nut is always sold shelled since the nut in the shell contains a toxin covering the actual nut.

Similar to the Brazil nut, cashews are not viewed as a Superfood Nut because of the higher saturated fat content and the lower unsaturated fat content. Few studies show any positive health benefits to cashews beyond the nutritional value they provide. The following shows the nutritional information for raw cashews.

Calories / 1 ounce serving 157
Protein (g) 5.2
Total Fat (g) 12.4
Saturated Fat (g) 2.2
Monounsaturated Fat (g) 6.7
Polyunsaturated Fat (g) 2.2
Carbohydrates (g) 8.6

Dietary Fiber (g) 0.9
Potassium (mg) 187
Magnesium (mg) 83
Zinc (mg) 1.6
Copper (mg) 0.6
Selenium (mcg) 6.6
Manganese (mg) 0.6
Vitamin B6 (mg) 0.1
Folate (mcg) 7
Riboflavin (mg) 0
Niacin (mg) 0.3
Alpha-tocopherol (mg) 0.3
Calcium (mg) 10
Iron (mg) 1.9

USDA Food Composition Databases. https://ndb.nal .usda.gov/ndb/foods/show/3645?manu=&fgcd=&ds=. Accessed June 26, 2016.

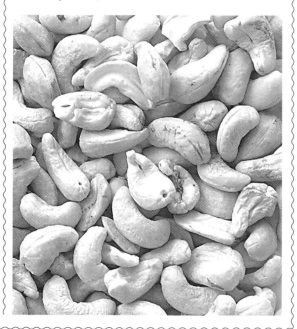

Cashews are an excellent source of copper, manganese, and magnesium and they are a good source of phosphorous, vitamin K, zinc, and iron. As with most nuts, cashews are a source of protein, which makes them a good snack option as well as a good alternative protein for those following a vegetarian eating plan.

HEALTH TIP: Cashews are commonly found in Asian dishes such as Cashew Chicken. If this dish is a favorite of yours, consider two adjustments to continue enjoying it. First, try preparing the dish at home and reduce the percent of calories from saturated fat by choosing white meat chicken, sautéing the chicken and vegetables in canola or olive oil, and by adding twice as many veggies as chicken and cashews. Second, if you enjoy this at your favorite Chinese restaurant, then balance the rest of your day with healthier fat choices.

HAZELNUTS

While you may not know as much about hazelnuts as some of the other Superfood Nuts, hazelnuts can use the qualified health claim (see Almonds). Hazelnuts, sometimes referred to as filberts, even though botanically the two are not the same, are rich in mono-unsaturated fat, the type often found in the Mediterranean diet. In addition, hazelnuts contain more polyunsaturated fat than saturated fat, making them good choices for aiding in the reduction of LDL cholesterol.

Calories / 1 ounce 178
Protein (g) 4.2
Total Fat (g) 17.2
Saturated Fat (g) 1.3
Monounsaturated Fat (g) 12.9
Polyunsaturated Fat (g) 2.2
Carbohydrates (g) 4.7
Dietary Fiber (g) 2.7
Potassium (mg) 193
Magnesium (mg) 46
Zinc (mg) 0.7
Copper (mg) 0.5
Selenium (mcg) 0.7
Manganese (mg) 1.7
Vitamin B6 (mg) 0.2
Folate (mcg) 32
Riboflavin (mg) 0
Niacin (mg) 0.5
Alpha-tocopherol (mg) 4.3
Calcium (mg) 32
Iron (mg) 1.3

USDA Food Composition Databases. https://ndb.nal.usda.gov/ndb/foods/show/3666?manu=&fgcd=&ds=. Accessed June 26, 2016.

Hazelnuts are an excellent source of manganese, copper, folate, and vitamin E and a good source of thiamin, magnesium, and fiber. Since nuts are plants, they contain a variety of phytonutrients (plant compounds), but the hazelnut has the highest amount of any nut of the phytonutrient proanthocyanidin. Proanthocyanidin is also found in cranberries, a food well known for its ability to help ward off urinary tract infections. Given the high amount of proanthocyanidin found in hazelnuts, they carry the same health benefit category as cranberries.

HEALTH TIP: Phytonutrients are plant compounds. "Phyto" in Greek means plant, and phytonutrients can help with disease prevention. They function as antioxidants, anti-inflammatories, and may act as anti-cancer agents. There are more than 25,000 phytonutrients in plant foods.

HEALTH TIP: Current dietary recommendations suggest that women under the age of 50 should aim for 25 grams of fiber per day and men under the age of 50 should aim for 38 grams of fiber per day. Recommendations for fiber intake drop after the age of 50 to 21 grams per day for women and 30 grams per day for men. Adequate fiber is important to digestive health, satiety, and possible maintenance of blood sugar and cholesterol levels. Remember, as you boost fiber intake you should also boost your fluid intake to avoid constipation that can occur with increased fiber intake. Current recommendations for fluid intake suggest that women consume at least 91 ounces a day and that men consume at least 125 ounces a day.

The Health and Medicine Division of the National Academies also states that all fluids, even those with caffeine, can count toward the daily fluid intake.

HEALTH TIP: Adequate folate, or folic acid, is important for all women of child-bearing age, even if they don't plan to get pregnant. Folate is important in the very early development of the neural tube, which eventually becomes the spinal cord and brain of the infant. Folate is found in most fruits and vegetables, and some nuts, but for most women of childbearing age to consume enough folate to aid in the prevention of spina bifida it is recommended that they consume 400 micrograms of folic acid from fortified grain foods, vitamin supplementation, or (more likely) a combination of the two.

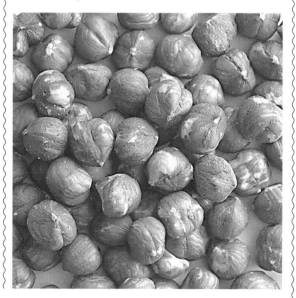

MACADAMIAS

Macadamias probably cause you to think about Hawaii, one of the main places where macadamias are produced, and for that reason they are often viewed as more of a delicacy. Macadamias are not viewed as a Superfood Nut for the same reason that the Brazil nut and cashews are not viewed as such: their fat content. Macadamias have the highest fat content of nuts, so they do not qualify for the qualified health claim. The high saturated fat content makes them a "use occasionally" nut.

Calories / 1 ounce 204
Protein (g) 2.2
Total Fat (g) 21.5
Saturated Fat (g) 3.4
Monounsaturated Fat (g) 16.7
Polyunsaturated Fat (g) 0.4
Carbohydrates (g) 3.9
Dietary Fiber (g) 2.4
Potassium (mg) 104
Magnesium (mg) 37
Zinc (mg) 0.4
Copper (mg) 0.2
Selenium (mcg) 3.3
Manganese (mg) 0.9
Vitamin B6 (mg) 0.1
Folate (mcg) 3
Riboflavin (mg) 0
Niacin (mg) 0.7
Alpha-tocopherol (mg) 0.2
Calcium (mg) 24
Iron (mg) 1.1

USDA Food Composition Databases. https://ndb.nal.usda.gov/ndb/foods/show/3673?manu=&fgcd=&ds=. Accessed June 26, 2016.

Macadamias are an excellent source of manganese and a good source of thiamin, having about 15 percent of the Daily Value. In addition to these two nutrients, macadamias are a good source of monounsaturated fats, coming in as the nut with the highest amount ounce for ounce.

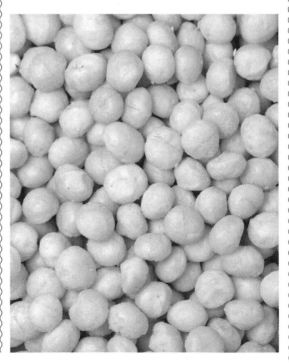

MONOUNSATURATED FATS

Monounsaturated fats are types of fat that seem to be beneficial in lowering the LDL cholesterol, thus lowering your risk for heart disease. The term "monounsaturated" refers to the chemical structure of the fat; and as you might have guessed, the prefix "mono" means there is one unsaturated bond in the molecule. While most foods that contain monounsaturated fatty acids also contain a mix of saturated and polyunsaturated fat, the important point in choosing fats is in choosing foods that provide a higher number of monounsaturated fatty acids, rather than saturated fatty acids. Monounsaturated fats are found in higher amounts in most nuts and nut butters; oils such as canola, olive, and peanut; avocados; and seeds.

PECANS

Pecans, like other nuts, are rich in phyto-nutrients and healthy monounsaturated fats. The phytonutrients in pecans can help protect against heart disease by preventing oxidation, or breakdown of LDL (bad) cholesterol. The monounsaturated fats in pecans also contribute to LDL reduction, making the pecan a double benefit for heart disease prevention.

In addition, pecans have been studied in connection with brain health and weight control. Recent studies have looked at the role pecans might play in helping to delay age-related motor neuron degeneration such as is found in those with Lou Gehrig's disease (also known as Amyotrophic Lateral Sclerosis, or ALS). The studies have looked at the vitamin E or tocopherol content of pecans as the possible connection. Vitamin E is an antioxidant that might help neurological function. The studies are still very preliminary, so whether pecans can truly help with this is not yet clear, but the nutrition in pecans can't hurt your overall diet.

In the studies on weight control, pecans, along with almonds and walnuts, seem to help boost metabolism, causing the body to burn more calories. But again, this is early research.

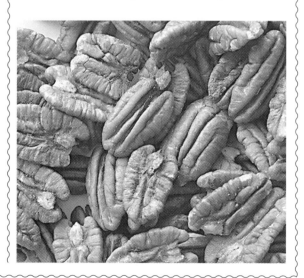

While the exact role pecans might play in health is not totally clear, what we do seem to know is that the nutrient package of pecans consists of a nice nutrient balance with no one nutrient outweighing another. It is an excellent source of manganese and a good source of copper, thiamin, and fiber.

Calories / 1 ounce 196
Protein (g) 2.6
Total Fat (g) 20.4
Saturated Fat (g) 1.8
Monounsaturated Fat (g) 11.6
Polyunsaturated Fat (g) 6.1
Carbohydrates (g) 3.9
Dietary Fiber (g) 2.7
Potassium (mg) 116
Magnesium (mg) 34
Zinc (mg) 1.3
Copper (mg) 0.3
Selenium (mcg) 1.1
Manganese (mg) 1.3
Vitamin B6 (mg) 0.1
Folate (mcg) 6
Riboflavin (mg) 0
Niacin (mg) 0.3
Alpha-tocopherol (mg) 0.4
Calcium (mg) 20
Iron (mg) 0.7

USDA Food Composition Databases. https://ndb.nal.usda.gov/ndb/foods/show/3681?manu=&fgcd=&ds=. Accessed June 26, 2016.

HEALTH TIP: Pecans are packed with plant sterols, a type of lipid that can work in the body to actually help lower blood cholesterol levels. While sterols have a similar chemical structure to cholesterol, they act in an entirely different way in the body. So instead of contributing to heart disease risk, they help with prevention. It is likely that their similar chemical structure to cholesterol helps them lower cholesterol. In the intestine, sterols likely block cholesterol absorption causing it to be excreted with other waste products. Add a few pecans to your morning oatmeal to get a double heart health benefit.

PINE NUTS

Pine nuts, also referred to as pignolis or piñons, provide a wide variety of nutrients and healthy fat but are probably best known for the manganese they contain. A one-ounce portion of pine nuts will provide 120 percent of the Daily Value for manganese. Manganese is a mineral that works with an antioxidant enzyme to help the body fight inflammation. In addition, pine nuts provide a good amount of copper, magnesium, and phosphorous. As with so many nuts, the fatty acid profile of pine nuts puts them in the favorable category for healthier fats.

Calories / 1 ounce 190

Protein (g) 4.0

Total Fat (g) 20.0

Saturated Fat (g) 1.5

Monounsaturated Fat (g) 5.5

Polyunsaturated Fat (g) 10.0

Carbohydrates (g) 4.0

Dietary Fiber (g) 1.0

Potassium (mg) 169

Magnesium (mg) 7.5

Zinc (mg) 1.9

Copper (mg) 0.4

Selenium (mcg) 0.2

Manganese (mg) 2.5

Vitamin B6 (mg) 0

Folate (mcg) 10.2

Riboflavin (mg) 0.07

Niacin (mg) 1.3

Alpha-tocopherol (mg) 2.8

Calcium (mg) 4.8

Iron (mg) 1.65

USDA Food Composition Databases. https://ndb.nal
.usda.gov/ndb/foods/show/3685?manu=&fgcd=&ds=.
Accessed June 30, 2016.

In addition to these nutrients, pine nuts contain the phytonutrient lutein and the polyunsaturated fat pinolenic acid. Lutein acts as other antioxidants in the body in promoting eye health, and pinolenic acid enhances the work of hormones, may play a role in satiety, and may help lower the LDL cholesterol.

There have been reports of a bitter taste occurring in the mouth after consuming pine nuts. The taste, similar to a metallic flavor, is reported to occur a few days after consumption. The FDA has reviewed complaints about "pine mouth" and has determined that it is an adverse food reaction but not a food allergy. Fortunately the symptoms last for a short period of time with no lingering impacts. The FDA continues to study this reaction to pine nuts to determine cause, severity of the symptoms, and any connections to a food allergy.

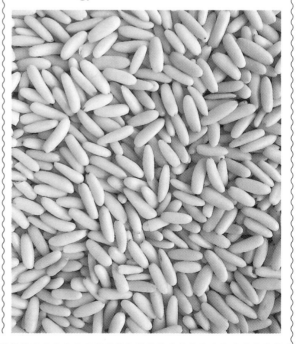

PISTACHIOS

Pistachios have the second highest polyphenol and flavonoid content, a fact that is visible when looking at their green color. In addition, they are a good source of the phytonutrients lutein and zeaxanthin, which help with eye health. Pistachios contain the highest amount of vitamin B6 of the nuts in this book, making them a beneficial food for keeping hormones balanced and healthy. Along with vitamin B6 pistachios provide almost three times the potassium of many other nuts. The pistachio is also a better source of fiber than many other nuts with only the almond coming in with a higher amount.

While those nutrients might be the "stars" of the pistachio, its overall nutrient package is very different from many other nuts. Pistachios have more carbohydrates than all nuts except for cashews, their fat content is the second lowest of all nuts, and they have the second highest polyunsaturated fat content.

Calories / 1 ounce 159
Protein (g) 5.8
Total Fat (g) 12.9
Saturated Fat (g) 1.6
Monounsaturated Fat (g) 6.8
Polyunsaturated Fat (g) 3.9

Carbohydrates (g) 7.8
Dietary Fiber (g) 2.9
Potassium (mg) 291
Magnesium (mg) 34
Zinc (mg) 0.6
Copper (mg) 0.4
Selenium (mcg) 2.6
Manganese (mg) 0.4
Vitamin B6 (mg) 0.5
Folate (mcg) 14
Riboflavin (mg) 0
Niacin (mg) 0.4
Alpha-tocopherol (mg) 0.7
Calcium (mg) 30
Iron (mg) 1.1

USDA Food Composition Databases. https://ndb.nal.usda.gov/ndb/foods/show/3687?manu=&fgcd=&ds=. Accessed June 30, 2016.

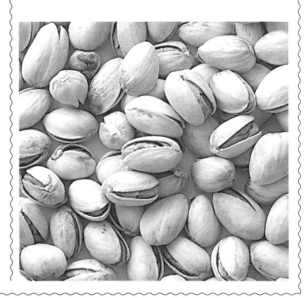

HEALTH TIP: Eating in-shell pistachios slows down the amount consumed because removing them from the shell takes time and allows you to recognize feelings of fullness and satisfaction sooner. In fact, studies have shown that eating in-shell pistachios reduces the number of calories consumed by about 40 percent compared to eating the pistachio kernels out of the shell. Awareness of what we are eating is an essential part of controlling calories.

HEALTH TIP: Americans struggle to consume enough potassium. Current guidelines suggest a daily intake of 4,700 milligrams, but the average daily intake is about half of that. Potassium helps the body regulate fluid balance, blood pressure, nerve impulses, and muscle contraction. Some studies indicate that lack of potassium might be as important, if not more important, to controlling blood pressure than sodium consumption.

Find potassium in most fruits and vegetables, fish, dairy, meat, and nuts. One ounce of pistachios has 291 milligrams of potassium, more than the amount found in a medium orange.

WALNUTS

Along with almonds, walnuts are probably the most studied nut, so more is known about their health benefits. Walnuts are the only nut that provides an excellent source of alpha-linolenic acid, which is the plant form of omega-3 fatty acid. The omega-3 fatty acid ALA is an essential fatty acid needed to help fight inflammation, aid in reduction of heart disease risk, prevent arrhythmias, and aid in prevention of blood clots. ALA can be converted by the body to EPA and DHA, two other omega-3's that function like ALA, but since they can be produced through ALA conversion, they are not essential fatty acids.

In addition to omega-3, walnuts have the highest antioxidant content of all the tree nuts. A study out of the University of Scranton actually commented about walnuts and their antioxidant content by stating "that an ounce of walnuts [has] more antioxidants than the sum of what

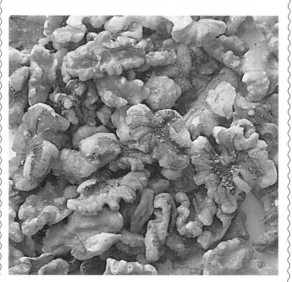

the average person consumes each day from fruits and vegetables." Another study found that walnuts are second only to blackberries in terms of their antioxidant content.

Research studies have looked at the health benefits of walnuts in the areas of heart health, cancer prevention, aging and cognitive function, diabetes, weight management, and male reproductive health.

When it comes to basic nutrients, walnuts are a source of quite a variety of nutrients but they are a good source of magnesium and phosphorous.

Calories / 1 ounce 190
Protein (g) 4.3
Total Fat (g) 18.0
Saturated Fat (g) 1.5
Monounsaturated Fat (g) 2.5
Polyunsaturated Fat (g) 13.4
Carbohydrates (g) 4.0
Dietary Fiber (g) 1.9
Potassium (mg) 125
Magnesium (mg) 45
Zinc (mg) 0.9
Copper (mg) 0.5
Selenium (mcg) 1.3
Manganese (mg) 0.95
Vitamin B6 (mg) 0.2
Folate (mcg) 28

Riboflavin (mg) 0
Niacin (mg) 0.3
Alpha-tocopherol (mg) 0.2
Calcium (mg) 28
Iron (mg) 0.8

USDA Food Composition Databases. https://ndb.nal.usda.gov/ndb/foods/show/3690?manu=&fgcd=&ds=h. Accessed July 8, 2016.

Walnuts provide an excellent source of gamma-tocopherol, a form of vitamin E that might be a part of why they are such strong anti-inflammatory nuts.

Walnuts also contain melatonin, which helps with sleep but might also be connected to some of the studies that show walnuts aid cognitive function and cancer prevention. Walnuts' main benefits are their heart healthy properties. Multiple studies continue to support that walnuts help lower both total cholesterol and LDL or bad cholesterol as well as blood pressure, and they increase HDL or good cholesterol and the health of blood vessels.

HEALTH TIP: Essential fatty acids are fats that cannot be made by the body but are needed for health. In addition to the omega-3 fatty acid, alpha-linolenic acid, the omega-6 fatty acid, or linoleic acid, is also an essential fatty acid. Linoleic acid is found in vegetable oils, nuts, seeds, and some animal foods. Essential fatty acids need to be consumed on a daily basis to meet the body's needs and aid the body in making other fatty acids.

HEALTH TIP: Omega-3 fatty acids are found in fatty fish, walnuts, flaxseeds, and chia seeds. The omega-3 in fatty fish is different from the plant sources of omega-3, but both forms seem to provide cardiovascular health benefits. Current recommendations suggest that we consume at least 6 ounces of fish per week and then add the plant sources of omega 3 to provide adequate intake. For those who follow a vegetarian or vegan eating plan, consuming adequate omega-3 from plant foods is especially important. Since omega-3 is limited to the foods listed above, those who follow a vegetarian or vegan eating plan need to find ways to include these foods routinely in order to consume enough omega-3.

HEALTH TIP: Vitamin E is a fat-soluble vitamin that works as an antioxidant, possibly helping to lower the risk for stroke and helping protect some of the essential fatty acids in foods. Vitamin E is found in most oils.

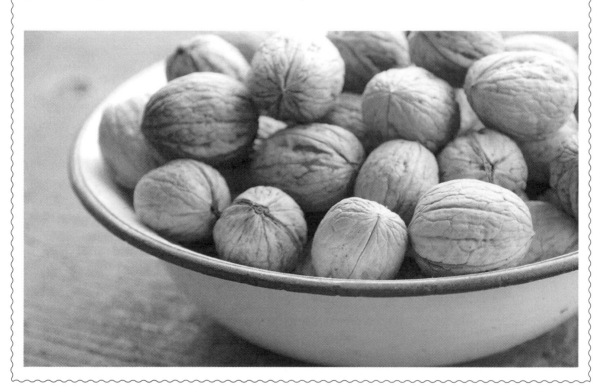

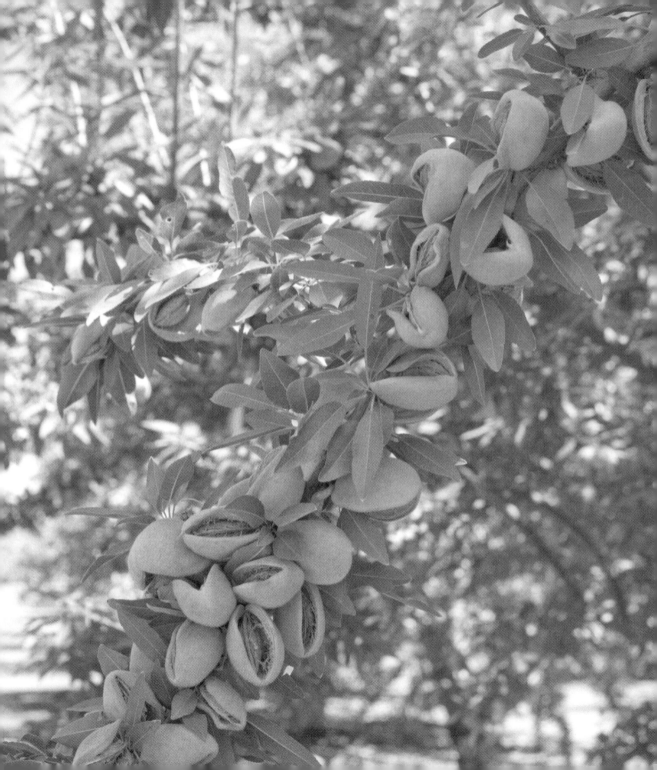

CHAPTER 2

HISTORY OF SUPERFOOD NUTS

M ost of us think about nuts in terms of snacks or maybe as a topping for another food or dish when, in fact, for centuries nuts have been a significant part of many cultures' diets.

Nuts, as defined in botany, are simply dried fruits with one seed enclosed in a tough outer layer. By that definition, true edible nuts are the chestnut and the hazelnut or filbert. But in culinary terminology, nuts are any large, oily seed found within a hard shell.

The term "Superfood Nuts" was coined to reflect the group of nuts that seem to provide a wide variety of health benefits. The prefix "super" can sometimes imply that foods carry almost magical benefits in and of themselves. While some nuts do exceed others in terms of health and nutritional benefits, no single food can meet all nutritional or health needs, so no one food is "super." Nevertheless, the knowledge of the nutritional benefits of nuts goes back in food history to many civilizations ago.

Evidence varies on how long nuts have been a part of food patterns, but a study from Hebrew University of Jerusalem in 2002

reported evidence indicating that 780,000 years ago, people in the area of modern-day Israel ate nuts. At a prehistoric dig, researchers found remains of nuts and stone tools used to crack them. Interestingly, the tools found at this site are similar to tools that archaeologists digging in Europe and North America found 4,000 to 8,000 years ago. In the report from Hebrew University of Jerusalem, seven types of nuts were found at the site: wild almond; prickly water lily or foxnut, which is no longer a nut we eat; two types of acorn; pistachio; Atlantic pistachio; and water chestnut. The Mediterranean is well known for nuts throughout culinary history.

Depending on which study you embrace, the oldest walnut usage, and possibly the oldest tree food, was found in 50,000 BCE in Iran. It is clear that walnuts were a frequently used crop in this part of the Middle East. The Romans viewed walnuts as food for the gods, often referring to them as "Jupiter's royal acorn." Walnuts were valued for their oil and were often used as a thickener, much as we use cornstarch today. Given the plentiful supply of walnuts and their value, they were commonly traded by English ships throughout the Mediterranean to other areas of the world leading to the development of the term "English walnuts." The English walnut is the one that was brought to California from Spain by the Franciscans in the late 1700s.

Almonds and pistachios are both mentioned in the Bible. While it is believed that almonds actually originated in China and Central Asia, they are more commonly mentioned in food patterns from Greece and other Mediterranean countries. The use of almonds at Roman wedding ceremonies, as a gift for long life, health, wealth, happiness, and fertility is a tradition still observed by many Italian families. Almonds also appeared, and continue to be used, in the sweet paste marzipan, a staple of Italian baking. Marzipan was brought to Europe by the Crusaders as early as the eleventh century, and in the 1800s royalty throughout Europe viewed it as a delicacy and a treat for special occasions.

The pistachio, like so many nuts, originated in the Middle East, with the most prevalent mentions of it in the area around Syria and Persia. Owning pistachio groves was viewed as a sign of wealth and conferred a high social status. Alexander the Great is thought to have been the transporter of pistachios to Greece during his conquests in 300 BCE. As the Roman Empire created its territory, consumption of pistachios spread to Italy and Spain. As pistachios traveled farther into Europe, they were added to baking traditions and viewed as a delicacy for the wealthy. In the 1880s pistachios were exported from Europe to the United States and were especially popular in areas where the Middle Eastern population was high. After World War I the pistachio was viewed as a more frequent or common snacking nut.

In 1929 an American botanist traveled to Persia, present day Iran, to collect pistachios with the intent of planting them in the central valley of California. Those early efforts at planting proved challenging, and only one seed actually developed into a tree. After years of experimenting, plants finally emerged in California in the 1960s. Pistachio trees are slow to yield fruit, requiring seven to ten years to mature, but in 1976 the first crop was available for sale in the US.

The pistachio is a member of the Anacardiaceae family, the same botanical family as the cashew. The cashew tree is native to northeastern Brazil and India but it likely arrived in Central America when Spanish sailors traveled there in the sixteenth century.

Later that century Portuguese missionaries took the nuts from Central America to East Africa and back to India. The preferred climate for the cashew is the low-altitude, moist, seacoast climate offered by countries such as Mozambique in Africa and Goa on the western shore of India. The cashew tree or shrub is an evergreen tree that produces oily nuts but also wood used for shipping crates and boats. Cashews are also used to make a gum that can be used for thickening, similar to gum arabic, the hardened sap of the acacia tree. The cashew nut is a bit different from other nuts in that it has two shells. The outer is smooth, thin, and somewhat elastic and of a greenish color until maturity, when it turns red. The inner shell is harder and must be cracked like other nuts, but in between the two shells is an oil that is similar to the toxic component of poison ivy and will irritate and blister human skin. This toxin is the reason that cashews are always sold shelled: to remove the toxic oil.

Not surprisingly, the Brazil nut is native to Brazil. Brazil nuts were first mentioned in 1569 when a Spanish officer fed them to his troops. The Dutch are credited with taking Brazil nuts to Europe in the late seventeenth century as a part of their trade missions. The Brazil nut grows well in most of South America, favoring the environment of the Amazon River basin.

Macadamias hail from southeastern Queensland, Australia. The macadamia, sometimes called the Australian nut, grows in rain forests and close to streams. In the early 1800s it was introduced to Hawaii, where it was basically an ornamental tree. Since then the nut has been cultivated in Brazil, regions of South Africa that offer moist mineral rich soil, and in areas of California that offer a similar soil composition. Macadamias grow on evergreen trees, the fruits resulting from white flowers that bloom in the summer. Although the trees are evergreens, the nuts prefer a milder, frost-free climate; still, some can survive in climates that experience occasional frosts. There are seven varieties of macadamias, but only two are edible. One is a smooth-shelled nut and the other has a rougher shell.

Sixteenth-century remnants of pecans have been found in archaeological excavations in northern Mexico and western Texas. One of the first known pecan trees was one planted by Spanish colonists and Franciscan monks. The word "pecan" comes from a Native American language and it means "all nuts requiring a stone to crack."

US colonists planted pecan trees in the late 1700s in New York and, following this, the trees appeared in gardens of many eastern US residents. George Washington and Thomas Jefferson are both known to have had pecan trees in their gardens. As the French and Spanish colonists realized the economic potential of pecans, exporting the crop became a priority. The Spanish colonists in Mexico exported the nut back to Spain in the early 1800s while the French started exporting from the Gulf of Mexico to the West Indies. As trade grew so, too, did the pecan industry, with orchards established from San Antonio across the Gulf Coast to South Carolina. In South Carolina a technique was discovered that allowed growers to graft plants to improve the yield. In 1876 the technique was perfected by a slave gardener in Louisiana and it is this grafting that vastly improved the crop and its yield. In North America pecans grow in Georgia, New Mexico, and Texas, as well as in Mexico.

For more than 10,000 years Native American tribes such as the Washo, Shoshone, Paiute, and Hopi used pine nuts as their main source of food. Pine nuts are found in pine trees that grow in the foothills of the Sierra Nevada range, coast of California, Great Basin, and Rocky Mountains down to Mexico. The trees grow in a variety of soils, resulting in varying tree heights and pine cone sizes. Pine nuts are found within the pine cone.

In addition to relying on the pine nut for food, Native Americans still dry the nuts to use as decorative beads or pulverize them to yield a salve used medicinally.

NUTS THROUGH THE YEARS

Nuts have been a part of eating plans for centuries, yet how they are included has changed over time. When people did more traveling on foot, nuts were a good choice as a meal or for snacking, given their portability. As availability of agriculture and cattle grew, nuts went from being a main ingredient to a supplemental component to nutrition.

In recent times nuts have served as afterschool snack options, baseball and football game treats, as a dish of nibbles when company came, and as a quick grab in the middle of the day. Nuts remained popular until in the 1970s when fat, types of fat, and the calories in fat became a concern.

As Americans moved away from active lifestyles, relied more on wheels than walking, and sat inside more than working outdoors, they experienced weight gain, and the fat and calories in nuts became focal points. In the 1980s food choices shifted from high-fat foods, no matter what their source, to foods that were low in fat and often low in calories. During this time nuts were foods for an occasional splurge, viewed as

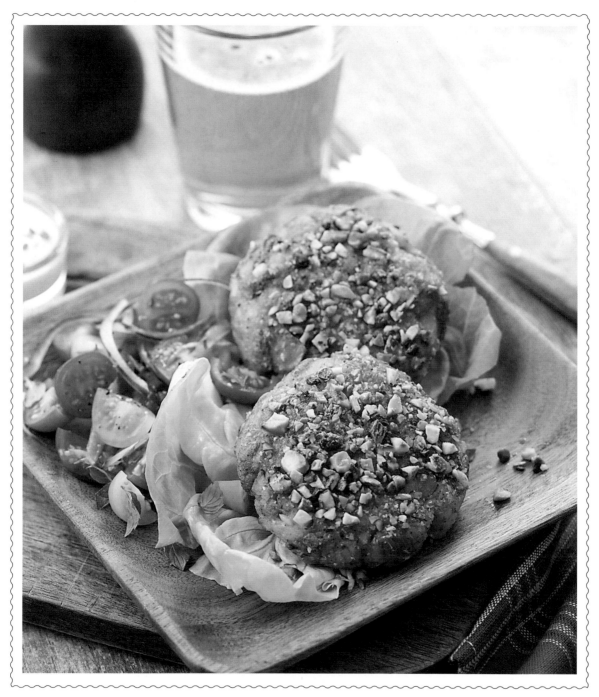

Curry Spiced Pistachio Crusted Potato Cakes, page 81

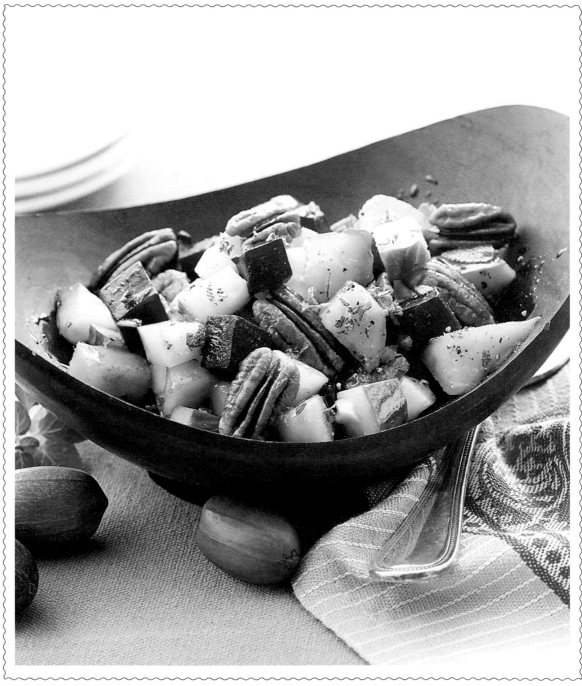

Beet and Pecan Salad with Mango and Cucumber, page 61

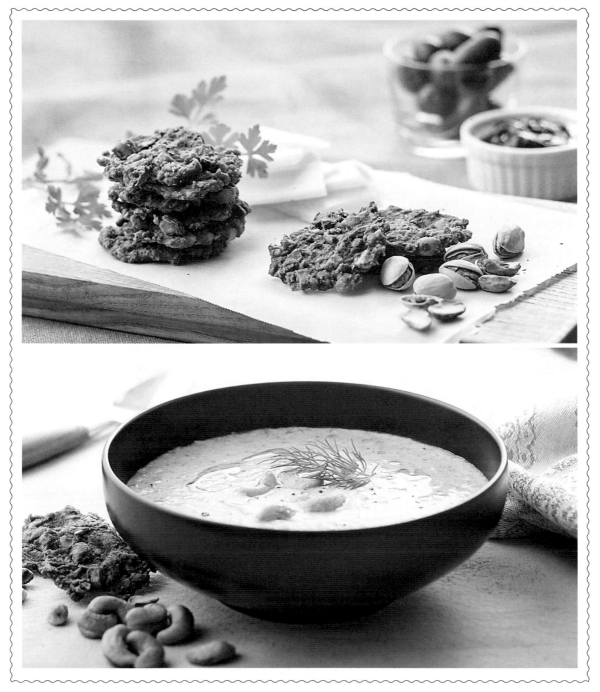

TOP: Pistachio Curry Crackers, page 102 BOTTOM: Bok Choy Cream Soup, page 53

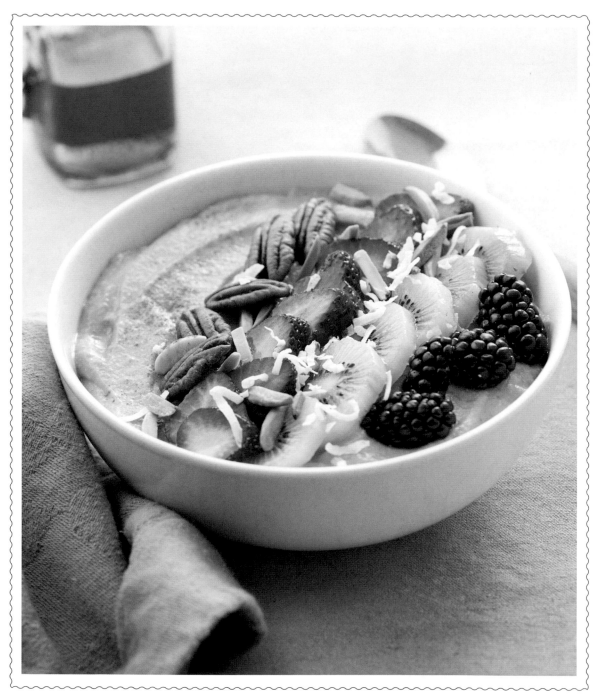

Sweet Tater Pie Smoothie Bowl, page 48

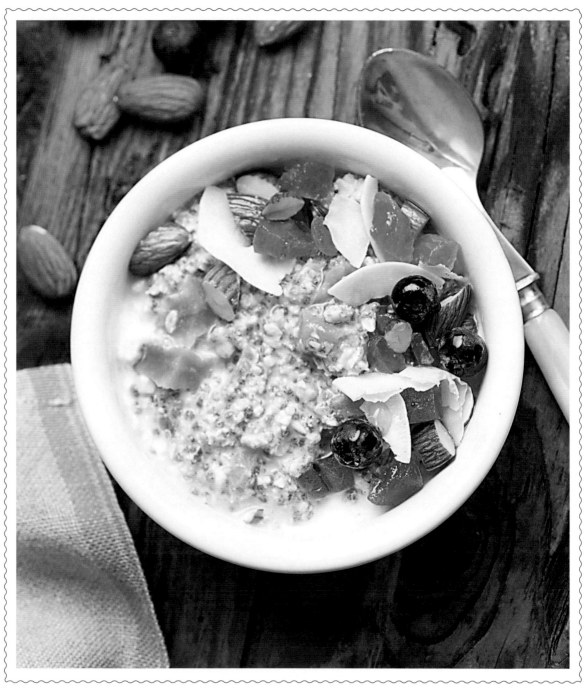

Almond Apricot Chia Muesli, page 34

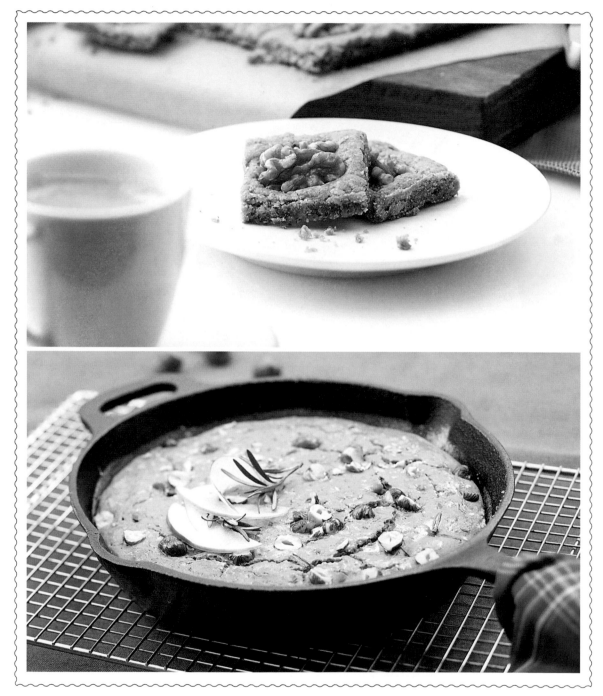

TOP: Maple Walnut Shortbread, page 112   BOTTOM: Hazelnut Rosemary Skillet Bread, page 100

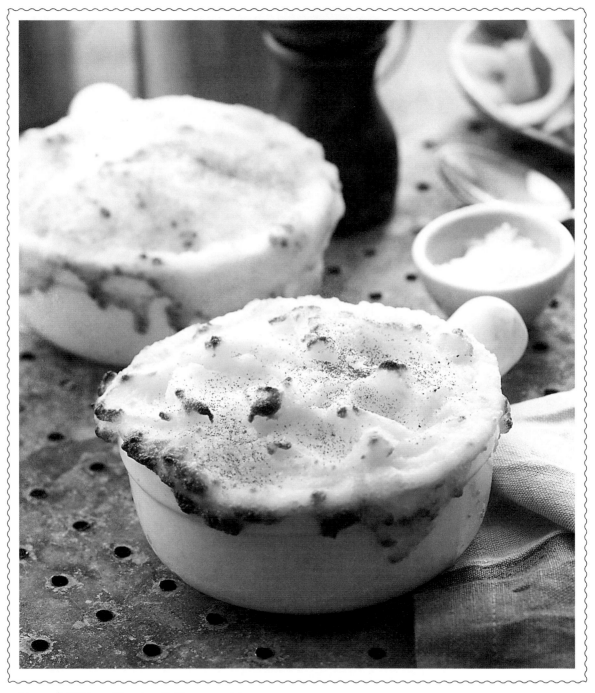

Tempeh Walnut Shepherd's Pie, page 88

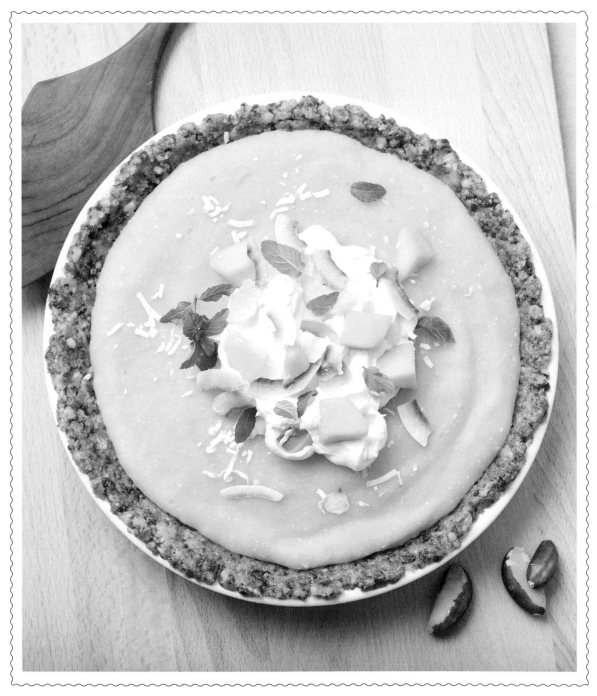

Mango Pie with Brazil Nut Crust, page 110

special-occasion treats and not things to be consumed daily.

While some health professionals still spoke of the nutritional value of nuts, their comments were always qualified with a "watch your portions" statement.

As research continued on the importance of fats in the diet and for health, conventional wisdom about nuts slowly improved, with interest in nuts as a part of a regular healthful eating plan finally becoming part of the *Dietary Guidelines for Americans*.

DIETARY GUIDELINES FOR AMERICANS

In 2010 the body of scientific evidence once again looked favorably on nuts and they were called out in the *Guidelines* with this statement: "For example, moderate evidence indicates that eating peanuts and certain tree nuts (i.e., walnuts, almonds, and pistachios) reduces risk factors for cardiovascular disease when consumed as part of a diet that is nutritionally adequate and within calorie needs."

The *Guidelines* also suggested that using nuts in place of animal protein could further help reduce the risk of heart disease and improve health. With this support, nuts regained favor as a mealtime option and a good choice for snacks. While the *Dietary Guidelines* did remind people that calories count and therefore nuts should be used within the scope of an individual's calorie allowance, meal plans were provided to help people learn how to do this. The evolving research with a variety of nuts, almonds, walnuts, and pistachios in particular, has made them "hot" in social media and therefore they have been recognized as something worth adding to meal plans. While some nuts have generated more interest than others, the market for nuts has escalated over the last several years.

From 2010 to 2015 the research on the health benefits of nuts grew significantly, as evidenced in chapter 1. The 2015 *Dietary Guidelines* included nuts in multiple chapters, in sample meal plans, and in a variety of amounts. The *Guidelines* talked about nuts in the same sentence as animal protein choices, demonstrating that nuts can provide the nutrient package we need and be a source of protein in just about any eating plan and can make variety in a vegetarian eating plan even better. In addition, the 2015 *Dietary Guidelines* committee looked at how our food choices impact the environment, and nuts were identified as a food that can help keep agriculture and land usage sustainable, thus supporting their inclusion in place of animal protein. The committee also addressed the wide body of evidence related to the healthy fat composition of nuts.

The 2015 *Dietary Guidelines* have put nuts back in the spotlight, and consumers are turning to them for quick meals and easy snack options, but nuts are also finding their way into salads, stuffing, smoothies, desserts, and almost every course on the menu, something you will see in the recipes in the book.

THE FUTURE OF NUTS

The current body of scientific evidence about the health benefits of nuts continues to grow, and many research studies on a variety of nuts are still ongoing. These studies likely mean that nuts will continue

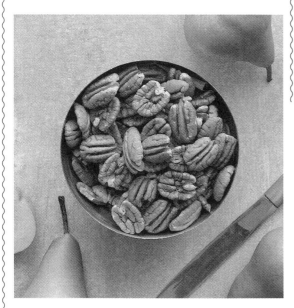

to be recognized as part of a healthy eating plan whether they're chosen as snacks or meals. As the research evolves it will be important to recognize that no single food is magic in terms of its health benefits, and no matter how super nuts might be, they still need to be combined with other foods to meet your nutrient needs. If your eating is currently built around animal protein choices, shifting to a healthier eating plan would mean adding a wide variety of fruits, vegetables and whole grains and choosing lean meat, fish, poultry, and low-fat or fat-free dairy. If you are a vegetarian or want to consume more plant-based protein options to meet your nutrient needs, you would want to add nuts to a good variety of fruits, vegetables, soy, and whole grains. So while this book focuses on the health benefits of nuts and identifies how they measure up as superfoods, don't forget the other foods that nuts need to partner with to make you super.

CHAPTER 3

BREAKFAST

Nuts are the perfect addition to a healthy, plant-based breakfast, making it sustaining and satisfying. They provide texture and the kind of nutrition that will quell the desire to snack before lunch. Breakfast around our house usually consists of fresh seasonal fruit and a grain—which is generally, but not always, rolled oats. It is served with soy milk and/or vegan yogurt and nuts.

Fruits are refreshing in the morning, offering natural sweetness that is delicious and appetizing. If you learn what grows in your area and when it is in season, and take the trouble to get it directly from the grower at your local farmers' market, you will be amazed at how good fresh fruit can be! I think we all have experienced tasteless out-of-season fruit that was picked too soon and kept too long, like the hard melon chunks served at most breakfast bars in hotels. For some people, this is their only experience of fresh fruit, which is a shame. Bananas are good, but get bold and add different fruits like mango, mulberry, and star fruit. Combine fresh, or even frozen fruit with a variety of grains and nuts, changing it around with the season, and your breakfast menu will never be dull. The combinations of fruits, nuts, and grains and what you can do with them are so numerous.

Mother Nature has the first say in the best breakfast menus, with stewed apples and hot porridge in the winter months and cold homemade cereal such as the Almond Apricot Chia Muesli (page 34) or Nutty Spicy Granola (page 39) in the summer. Since fruits in season change throughout the year, there is always a delectable variety of healthy breakfast options available. Pancakes are a great weekend treat all year round, and don't forget whole-grain toast with nut butter and fresh fruit, or one of the muffin recipes or breads in the Baked Goods chapter with a smoothie. These are the types of breakfasts that are worth waking up for!

ALMOND APRICOT CHIA MUESLI

MAKES 4 SERVINGS

Almonds and apricots combine beautifully in this delicious and nutritious muesli. You can make this the night before and keep it refrigerated until morning, or make it first thing in the morning, but it's best when it has soaked for at least 30 minutes before eating.

1¼ cups rolled oats

½ cup dried apricots

⅓ cup almonds

¼ cup chia seeds

1 teaspoon cinnamon

3 cups water, soy milk, or other vegan milk, or a combination

1 teaspoon vanilla extract

¼ teaspoon almond extract

1. Place the oats, apricots, and almonds in a blender and coarsely grind. Transfer to a mixing bowl.

2. Add the chia seeds and cinnamon. Mix well, then add the water or milk and the vanilla and almond extracts. Mix again and let set for at least 30 minutes.

3. Transfer to serving bowls, top with fresh fruit, and serve with vegan yogurt or milk.

ORANGE WALNUT MUESLI

MAKES 2 TO 3 SERVINGS

The orange zest in this cereal makes it deliciously refreshing and a great change from the usual. Serve it with whatever fresh fruit you have on hand: orange segments, sliced bananas, grated apples, fresh or frozen berries, mango chunks—anything!

½ cup rolled oats

2 tablespoons raisins

2-inch-square piece orange peel

½ cup walnut halves

2 tablespoons ground flaxseeds

⅔ cup orange juice

1 cup unsweetened soy milk, or other vegan milk

Fresh seasonal fruit

1. Combine the oats, raisins, and orange peel in a blender and grind. Then add the walnuts and coarsely grind.

2. Transfer the mixture to a bowl and add the ground flaxseeds. Mix well and add the orange juice and milk. Mix again and let set for at least 10 minutes.

3. Transfer the mixture to serving dishes, top with fresh fruit, and serve with more milk.

BREAKFAST RICE PUDDING

MAKES 2 SERVINGS

This nourishing breakfast uses up leftover cooked rice. Because turmeric is said to have therapeutic anti-inflammatory properties, I sometimes like to see how much I can get into a recipe without turning it too bitter. To me, this tasted wonderful with 2 tablespoons of freshly grated turmeric. There is just 1 tablespoon in the recipe, though, but if you are open to experimenting and like the flavor, try adding up to 2 tablespoons. If you can't find fresh turmeric, start with ½ teaspoon turmeric powder.

1 teaspoon coconut oil

1 tablespoon fresh grated turmeric root

1 tablespoon fresh grated ginger root

1 cinnamon stick

6 cloves

½ teaspoon ground coriander

¼ teaspoon ground cardamom

1 medium apple, peeled, cored, and diced (leave peel on if organic)

1 cup cooked brown rice

2 cups unsweetened vegan milk

½ teaspoon vanilla extract

½ cup raisins

¼ cup pistachios

1. Heat the coconut oil in a medium-size saucepan. Add the turmeric and ginger, stir over medium heat for a minute, then add the rest of the spices and the apple. Stir again and add the rice. Mix well.

2. Stir in the milk and vanilla, and bring the mixture to a simmer, while continuing to stir. Cover, reduce the heat to low, and cook, stirring occasionally, for about 15 minutes, or until the apple is done and most of the milk has been absorbed.

3. Serve warm or cold with raisins, pistachios, and fresh seasonal fruit.

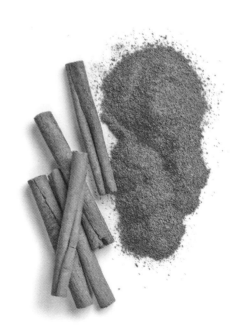

CRANBERRY PECAN PORRIDGE

MAKES 3 TO 4 SERVINGS

There is something so good about cranberries and pecans that you don't want to save the combo for Thanksgiving. This is best simmered slowly over low heat, but doesn't need much attention.

2 medium Pink Lady apples, diced
½ cup fresh or frozen cranberries
½ cup old-fashioned rolled oats
¼ cup raisins
2¼ cups water
1 cinnamon stick
6 cloves
1 tablespoon grated orange zest
½ cup chopped pecans

1. Place all the ingredients, except for the pecans, in a medium-size saucepan. Cover and bring to a simmer, then reduce the heat to low and cook, stirring occasionally, for about 20 minutes, or until the apples are cooked.

2. Transfer the porridge to serving bowls and top with the pecans. Serve with vegan yogurt or milk.

CEREAL TOPPING

MAKES ABOUT 3 CUPS

This is a tasty topping to sprinkle on porridge and it can be blended together and stored in the refrigerator. I almost always have some on hand. The recipe is easy to cut in half, but it will keep nicely for about a month.

1 cup whole flaxseeds
½ cup almonds
¼ cup walnut halves
¼ cup pecans
2 tablespoons cinnamon

1. Place the flaxseeds in a blender and grind to a fine meal. Do this in two batches, if necessary. Transfer to a quart jar or other container.

2. Place the almonds in the blender and blend just enough to coarsely grind, then add them to the flaxseed.

3. Coarsely grind the walnuts and pecans together and add to the other ingredients. Add the cinnamon to the jar, or other container, with the flaxseed and shake or stir to mix. Cover and store. Use a tablespoon or two per serving over cooked porridge or fruit.

HAZELNUT PANCAKES

MAKES 4 TO 6 SERVINGS (ABOUT 28 PANCAKES)

These delicate pancakes are absolutely delicious! The garbanzo flour, soy milk, and ground hazelnuts make them a good source of protein, and they are so rich and flavorful that you don't need butter or syrup. Try them with stewed apples and fresh fruit.

½ cup hazelnuts

1 cup whole grain spelt flour

½ cup garbanzo flour

1½ teaspoons baking powder

½ teaspoon baking soda

2 cups unsweetened soy milk, or other vegan milk

2 tablespoons cider vinegar or balsamic vinegar

Olive oil for cooking, as needed

1. Place the hazelnuts in a blender or food processor and blend to a coarse meal. Transfer the nut meal to a large mixing bowl.

2. Add the spelt flour, garbanzo flour, baking powder, and baking soda to the mixing bowl and stir to combine well.

3. In a smaller bowl, combine the milk and vinegar. Stir.

4. Add the liquid to the mixing bowl with the dry ingredients and mix to form a batter.

5. Heat about 1 tablespoon of olive oil in a cast-iron or ceramic non-stick skillet. Drop about ¼ cup batter at a time onto the hot skillet. Cook 4 pancakes at a time over medium-high heat for 2 to 3 minutes, or until they are brown on the bottom. Flip them over and cook briefly until done. Serve immediately.

6. Transfer cooked pancakes to a 200°F oven to keep them warm until you get them all cooked.

TIP: To scoop up the batter for pancakes, I use a ¼-cup measuring cup with a handle. This way the pancakes are all about the same size.

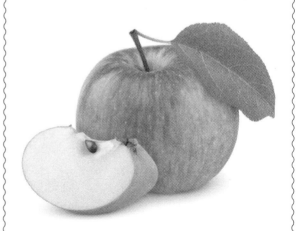

TEFF CHOCOLATE ALMOND PANCAKES

MAKES 4 TO 6 SERVINGS
(ABOUT 28 PANCAKES)

These pancakes are crisp around the edges and full of rich chocolaty flavor and nutty texture. They are perfect for weekend breakfast or brunch served with fresh fruit and unsweetened vegan yogurt, and you won't even miss butter or syrup!

½ cup almonds

1 cup teff flour

½ cup garbanzo flour

⅓ cup cocoa powder

2 teaspoons baking powder

½ teaspoon baking soda

1½ cups soy milk, or other vegan milk

2 tablespoons cider vinegar

Coconut oil, as needed

1. Place the almonds in a blender or food processor and blend to a coarse meal. Transfer the nut meal to a large mixing bowl.

2. Add the two flours, cocoa powder, baking powder, and baking soda to the mixing bowl with the almond meal. Mix well.

3. In a smaller bowl, combine the milk and vinegar. Stir.

4. Add the liquid to the mixing bowl with the flour mixture. Mix well to form a fairly thick batter.

5. Heat about 1 tablespoon of coconut oil in a well-seasoned cast-iron or ceramic non-stick skillet. Drop about ¼ cup batter at a time onto the hot skillet. Cook 4 pancakes at a time over medium-high heat for 3 to 4 minutes, or until they are crispy and brown on the bottom and starting to dry out on the top. Flip them over and cook for 1 to 2 minutes, or until done.

6. Transfer cooked pancakes to a 200°F oven to keep them warm until you get them all cooked.

NOTE: For a fun and filling dessert (or even dessert for dinner if you're not too hungry and want something that seems decadent but isn't really), try a scoop of Easy Banana Pecan Nice Cream (see page 117) between two hot pancakes and top with a drizzle of chocolate sauce.

TIP: To speed up the pancake cooking process, make the fruit salad, stewed apples, sauce, or anything that you want to serve with the pancakes first, and then have two skillets going at the same time.

NUTTY SPICY GRANOLA

MAKES ABOUT 5 CUPS

You can make this granola and store it away in the refrigerator for when you want a hearty, high-energy breakfast or snack. It is crisp, not too sweet, and deliciously flavored, and I don't think anyone will know it is made with olive oil.

4 cups rolled oats

1 cup walnuts

1 tablespoon cinnamon

1 tablespoon ground ginger

1 teaspoon ground cardamom

½ cup olive oil

⅓ cup maple syrup

2 teaspoons vanilla extract

1. In a large mixing bowl, combine all the ingredients.

2. Spread the mixture out onto a single layer on a baking sheet.

3. Bake at 350°F for about 10 minutes. Remove from the oven and stir. Return to the oven and bake another 10 minutes. Remove from the oven and stir.

4. If the granola is not dry, which it probably will not be, return it to the oven with the oven turned off. Let it set in the hot oven for another 10 minutes or so until it is crisp and dry.

5. Let cool completely before storing in an airtight container or bag. It gets crisper as it cools.

NOTE: Add dried date pieces, raisins, or other dried fruit after the granola is done, if you want a sweeter cereal.

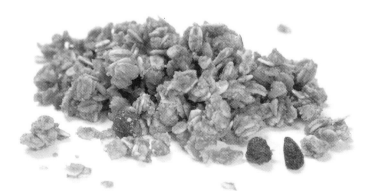

REMOVING THE SKIN FROM ALMONDS

There are two methods of skinning almonds—blanching and soaking. For milk, soaking is better because it softens the nuts. In a pinch Almond Milk will work with blanched unsoaked almonds, but you may have to blend the slurry a bit longer.

BLANCHING

Place as many almonds as you want to blanch in a bowl.

Bring enough water to cover the almonds to a rolling boil.

Pour the water over the almonds.

Let the almonds soak in the hot water for 1 minute.

Drain the almonds in a strainer and rinse with cool water.

Press each nut between your thumb and forefinger and the skin will easily slip off.

SOAKING

Soak the almonds covered in water for 8 hours, or up to overnight.

In the morning, drain and rinse the almonds.

Press each nut between your thumb and forefinger and the skin will easily slip off.

BASIC ALMOND MILK

MAKES 3½ TO 4 CUPS

Almond milk is so easy to make that there is no real need to buy it. Except for the soaking, it takes about 15 minutes from start to cleanup, and you control the quality of the ingredients. Also, there is the benefit of the leftover almond pulp that you can use in recipes. Some recipes call for soaking up to 2 days in the refrigerator, which you can do. Soaking them just 4 hours makes very nice milk; however, 8 to 10 hours of soaking does seem to make the milk slightly creamier.

Some recipes call for leaving the skin on the almonds, but I prefer to remove it before making the milk because I think the flavor is better, and the leftover white pulp is so good for making the Faux Chèvre Frais spread (page 43)! In fact, I like the faux chèvre so much that I do not press all the liquid out of the nuts in order to have more and creamier pulp to make the spread with.

EQUIPMENT
Blender

Colander or strainer

Mixing bowl

Clean cotton dishtowel—You can buy special nut milk bags, but I always make do with what I have on hand, and a dishtowel or linen napkin works perfectly well. A plain, white, cotton chef's towel is better than terrycloth, though. To clean it up afterward, just shake it outside then throw it in the wash.

1 cup almonds

4 cups water

1. Place the almonds in a small bowl and add water to cover and soak.

2. After soaking, remove the skins from the nuts by squeezing each one between your thumb and forefinger. The skin will slip right off.

3. Place the almonds in a blender with the water. If you have a small blender, you don't have to add all the water at once. Just add about 2 cups or enough to make a slurry that is easy to blend. Blend for about 3 minutes on high speed.

4. Line the colander with a clean dishtowel and place it inside a large bowl. Pour the slurry onto the towel. If you did not blend all the water with the almonds, you can add it now, pouring it onto the cloth.

5. Take the colander out of the bowl, then the towel out of the colander, and, holding the towel over the bowl, squeeze the almond slurry through the towel.

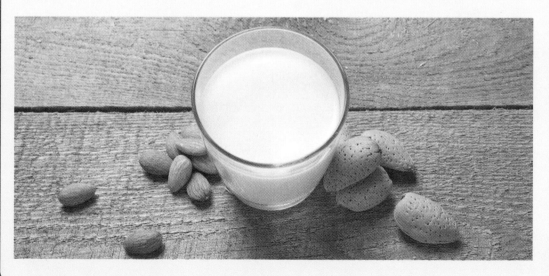

Squeeze and twist the towel until you have about 4 cups of milk.

6. Pour the milk into a jar with a lid. Homemade almond milk will last 3 to 4 days in the refrigerator.

FLAVOR OPTIONS: The flavor is great when it is plain, but you can add your choice of any of the following flavors or a combination of them:

½ teaspoon vanilla extract
Pinch of nutmeg
½ teaspoon cinnamon
1 date, blended into the milk
1 tablespoon maple syrup or coconut nectar

TIP: You can save time by buying blanched almonds, but I have found that sometimes they are not as fresh as the ones with the skin. It takes 5 to 10 minutes to remove the skin from a cup of soaked almonds, so if you are going to bother to make your own milk, it is probably worth it to skin the almonds yourself.

ALMOND CREAM

Use this recipe when you want something richer and creamier than almond milk. Simply follow the directions for Almond Milk, but decrease the quantity of water to 2 cups. To have the option of both Almond Cream and Almond Milk from one batch, start with Almond Cream and dilute it as needed for milk.

WHAT TO DO WITH THE LEFTOVER ALMOND PULP

If you squeeze the pulp down to extract as much milk as possible, there will be about ¼ cup pulp left in the towel. This can be added to cookies, muffins, porridge, muesli, smoothies, pancakes, crackers, and veggie burgers.

The Faux Chèvre Frais (facing page) can also work with only ¼ cup pulp, but it's not as creamy as it is with wetter pulp. If you want to make the faux chèvre, stop when you have about ½ cup to 1 cup pulp and you will have a nice consistency to make the spread.

FAUX CHEVRE FRAIS

MAKES ONE SMALL ROUND
ABOUT 2 INCHES IN DIAMETER
AND 1 INCH THICK

If you avoid dairy for any reason, it's worth it to make your own almond milk just so you can have this! It actually looks like a small round of fresh goat cheese. The texture is similar, too. If you serve it with some really good crackers without telling anyone except the vegans what it is, it will be gone before anyone questions it! This should be made from skinned almonds that have been soaked for 8 to 10 hours. It will not work if the skin is left on the nuts. The two recipes below are similar, but with different seasonings. I couldn't decide which one to use, so I used both!

DILL CHEVRE

Almond pulp left over from making milk
(about ½ cup)

1 tablespoon lemon juice or less, to taste

2 tablespoons mild olive oil

⅛ teaspoon salt, or to taste

1 small clove garlic, pressed

1 tablespoon minced dill weed

TRUFFLE GARLIC CHIVE CHEVRE

Almond pulp left over from making milk
(about ½ cup)

1 tablespoon or less white wine vinegar (if you
have truffle vinegar, use it)

2 tablespoons truffle olive oil

⅛ teaspoon salt, or to taste

1 clove garlic, pressed

1 tablespoon minced garlic chives, or chives

1. Place the almond pulp in a small bowl and mix in the lemon juice (or vinegar, for the Truffle version), olive oil, salt, and garlic.

2. Shape into a small patty. Place the minced herbs on a small plate and press into the round.

ALMOND YOGURT

Delicious yogurt can be made from homemade almond milk and a purchased culture (see Additional Resources on page 142). It will not be as thick as dairy yogurt, so many recipes use agar, arrowroot, or pectin to thicken it. Some use gelatin, but since gelatin is not vegan, I don't use it. I have used pectin, though, and found that following the recipe made the yogurt too thick, so I halved the quantity of pectin. There are several companies that sell yogurt cultures, so it is best to follow the recipe that comes with the culture you purchase.

HAZELNUT MILK

MAKES ABOUT 3 CUPS

Hazelnut Milk and Hazelnut Cream (see below) each have a marvelous flavor. Don't try to skin the nuts before making the milk, though, because it is not as easy to remove as almond skin. I think it is good with a little less water than is called for in Almond Milk.

1 cup hazelnuts

3 cups water

Soak the hazelnuts overnight and follow the steps for Almond Milk, omitting step two.

HAZELNUT CREAM

In the recipe above, substitute 2 cups of water.

GOLDEN MILK

MAKES 2 SERVINGS

Not only is this a delicious way to use nut milk, it contains spices that, in the ancient practice of Ayurveda, are considered therapeutic, anti-inflammatory, and warming. A nice hot mug of Golden Milk will help you to feel warm if you are fighting off a cold and feel chilled. The coconut oil is said to allow the turmeric to be better absorbed by the body. Honey is not vegan, but my personal feeling is that small local beekeepers do more to help than to hurt the bees. If you prefer, you can use another sweetener to replace the honey. In India, jaggery, a traditional unrefined sugar, would be used.

1 teaspoon coconut oil

1½-inch piece fresh turmeric root, cut into thin strips

½-inch piece fresh ginger root, cut into thin strips

1 cinnamon stick

8 cloves

6 cardamom pods, crushed

Freshly ground black pepper, to taste

1¾ cups water

1 cup almond milk or hazelnut milk

2 teaspoons raw local honey, to taste, or other sweetener

Pinch of cinnamon or ground nutmeg

1. In a saucepan, heat the oil and add the spices. Stir and let cook for a minute, then add the water. Cover and bring to a simmer. Simmer over low heat for about 10 minutes.

2. Add the milk and heat again until pleasantly warm to drink—it's not necessary to boil. Remove the pan from the heat and stir in the honey. Strain the mixture into serving mugs and top with a sprinkle of cinnamon or nutmeg.

NOTE: Peeling the ginger and turmeric is not necessary.

ALMOND CHAI

Follow the recipe for Golden Milk, but after the spices have boiled, add 2 heaping teaspoons black, loose-leaf tea. Let steep for 3 to 4 minutes and add the milk. Then reheat, add honey, and strain.

For cold chai, chill the mixture after adding the honey.

SMOOTHIES

Smoothies are easy and delicious. No wonder they are so popular! They are also a great way to get fruits and vegetables into people who otherwise might not have the time or inclination to eat those foods. I believe the reason for this is because smoothies are so enjoyable to drink. It's always easier to find time for something we like!

These simple recipes do not always contain the most obvious ingredient choices. The reason for this is to get a variety of healthy produce into your diet. Some recipes may contain ingredients you haven't thought of. Cucumber, for example, is a great choice for smoothies because it is so mild. Other mild-flavored vegetables such as spinach, fennel, and romaine lettuce are good, too. Just for fun, and because

I had some, I wanted to see if it was possible to make a good smoothie with radicchio. It was, as you will discover in the Trying Is Believing Pink Smoothie! There are lots of smoothie possibilities out there, and if you want to get more creative, check out the smoothie tips at the end of the chapter.

As with the other recipes in this book, these smoothies are not too sweet. More is not necessarily better when it comes to sweeteners and your health. Therefore, these recipes are sweet enough to be delicious, but not sweeter than need be. That said, I tested these recipes with the flavorful bananas from my garden, which are probably sweeter than the store-bought varieties. So if you need more sweetener in your smoothie, just add a soft pitted date or two or a few drops of stevia to the blender.

BLUEBERRY WALNUT SMOOTHIE

MAKES ABOUT 2 CUPS

Who says a recipe must be complicated to be good? Sometimes the simplest recipes are the best. This smoothie is full of nutrition and goodness and can be thrown together in a minute!

1 cup fresh blueberries
1 cup unsweetened soy milk, or nut milk
¼ cup walnuts
½ to 1 frozen peeled banana

1. Place all ingredients in a blender and blend until smooth.

2. Serve immediately. Enjoy!

VARIATIONS: Use any berry in place of the blueberries.

CHOCOLATE PECAN SMOOTHIE

MAKES ABOUT 2 CUPS

Breakfast, snack, or dessert—whenever you serve it, this smoothie is a delight! It tastes sweet, rich, and scrumptious, but it does not contain added sugar or extracted fat.

2 frozen bananas

3 tablespoons cocoa powder

½ teaspoon vanilla extract

1½ cups unsweetened soy milk, or nut milk

¼ cup pecans

1. Place all the ingredients in a blender and blend until smooth.

2. Serve immediately and enjoy!

VARIATION: This is a good recipe for experimenting with the quantity of milk. Make the smoothie thick enough to eat with a spoon by adding less milk, or thin enough to drink with a straw by adding more milk.

DELICIOUS GREEN SMOOTHIE

MAKES ABOUT 3 CUPS

This smoothie is a beautiful shade of green. Who would have thought that healthy veggies could be so delicious!

1½ cups pineapple cubes

1 cup baby spinach

½ medium cucumber, in thick slices

½ cup chopped fennel bulb

1 frozen banana

¼ cup walnuts

¾ cup water, apple juice, or pineapple juice

½ teaspoon vanilla extract

1. Place all ingredients in a blender and blend until smooth.

2. Enjoy immediately!

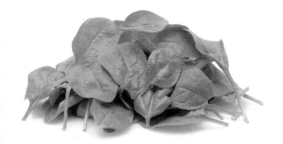

DELICIOUS RED SMOOTHIE

MAKES ABOUT 2 CUPS

The ginger, clove, and orange give this smoothie a complex and spicy flavor that takes your attention away from the beet and kale.

1 cup fresh orange juice

1 square inch organic orange peel

2 to 3 leaves red kale, stems removed

1 cup halved and hulled strawberries

1 small beet (about ⅔ cup diced)

1 frozen banana

¼ cup pecans

½ to 1 inch chunk of fresh ginger

3 to 4 cloves

1. Place all the ingredients in a blender and blend until smooth.

2. Enjoy immediately!

NOTE: When using citrus peel in recipes, make sure it is organic, because pesticides are absorbed into the skin of citrus.

LEMONY GREEN DELIGHT

MAKES ABOUT 3 CUPS

Light and refreshing, this smoothie gets a whole cucumber plus 2 cups spring mix into the glass. The color is beautiful and the taste is wonderfully lemony!

1 cup water or apple juice

1 small to medium cucumber, in thick slices

2 cups spring mix greens

2 frozen bananas

Juice of one lemon

Peel from ¼ lemon

⅓ cup walnuts

1. Place all the ingredients in a blender and blend until smooth.

2. Enjoy immediately!

TRULY TROPICAL TREAT

MAKES ABOUT 2 CUPS

You will not want to add kale or any other vegetable to this luscious smoothie. It is a pure and simple delight, like a mango lassi but without the sugar or dairy!

1 small to medium ripe mango

1 small frozen banana

1 cup water

¼ cup macadamia nuts

½ teaspoon vanilla extract

1. Place all the ingredients in a blender and blend until smooth.

2. Enjoy immediately!

TRYING IS BELIEVING PINK SMOOTHIE

MAKES ABOUT 3½ CUPS

I was able to get a whole cup of chopped radicchio and half of a cucumber into this smoothie without it tasting bitter or turning gray! If you don't believe me, try it!

1 cup chopped radicchio

1 cup sliced cucumber

1 cup halved and hulled strawberries

1 peach, pitted

1 frozen banana

½ cup unsweetened soy milk, or nut milk

¼ cup walnuts

1. Place all the ingredients in a blender and blend until smooth.

2. Enjoy immediately!

SMOOTHIE BOWL

Smoothie bowls are all the rage on Instagram. A smoothie bowl is simply a thick smoothie that you eat with a spoon rather than drink. You can make smoothie bowls by adding a handful of rolled oats to the blender, or a tablespoon or so of chia seeds, a couple of tablespoons of flaxseeds, or by reducing the liquid in a recipe.

To make your smoothie bowl attractive, top it with any fresh fruit you happen to have on hand. It's hard to go wrong here. For fun, you can swirl two different contrasting colors together, or make layers in a parfait glass.

SWEET TATER PIE SMOOTHIE BOWL

MAKES ABOUT 2 CUPS

Ever have sweet potato pie? Here it is in a bowl, but without the bad fat and sugar! To make it into a smoothie to drink in a glass, just use a half rather than a whole sweet potato.

1 cup vegan milk

1 small to medium baked sweet potato

¼ cup pecans or walnuts

1 tablespoon minced ginger

½ teaspoon ground cinnamon

3 cloves

¼ teaspoon vanilla extract

1. Place all the ingredients in a blender and blend until smooth.

2. Pour into one or two bowls, depending on how hungry you are. Top with a sprinkling of granola and some fresh fruit and enjoy immediately!

SMOOTHIE TIPS

- Adjust the liquid to make a smoothie thicker, to eat with a spoon, or thinner, to drink with a straw. The consistency of a smoothie will depend on many factors, so adjust the milk to your taste.

- The size for the bananas used in a smoothie makes a big difference as to its texture and sweetness, so feel free to add more or less banana to taste.

- Flaxseed or chia seeds thicken a smoothie a lot because of their mucilaginous qualities. Nuts will thicken a smoothie, too, but not nearly as much.

- Cucumber, some fruits, and certain leafy greens contain lots of water, so a smoothie will need less liquid when you use watery fruit and vegetables.

- If a smoothie is not sweet enough, add a soft pitted date or two, a few drops of stevia, or more banana or other sweet fruit.

- Vegetables that go well in fruit smoothies include romaine and iceberg lettuce, leaf lettuce, spinach, kale, cucumbers, sweet bell peppers, summer squash, parsley, fennel, celery, jicama, baked winter squash, and sweet potato—and you may be able to come up with more.

- You can always make a smoothie taste better by adding more fruit if it has become bitter because of too many vegetables!

- Nuts, hemp seeds, and bananas all add creaminess to a smoothie.

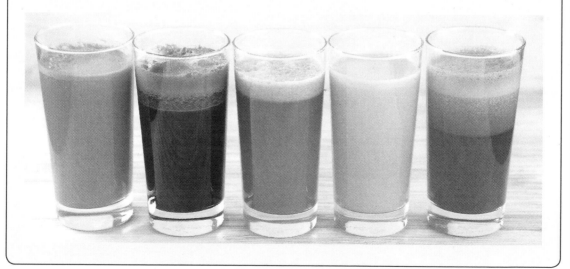

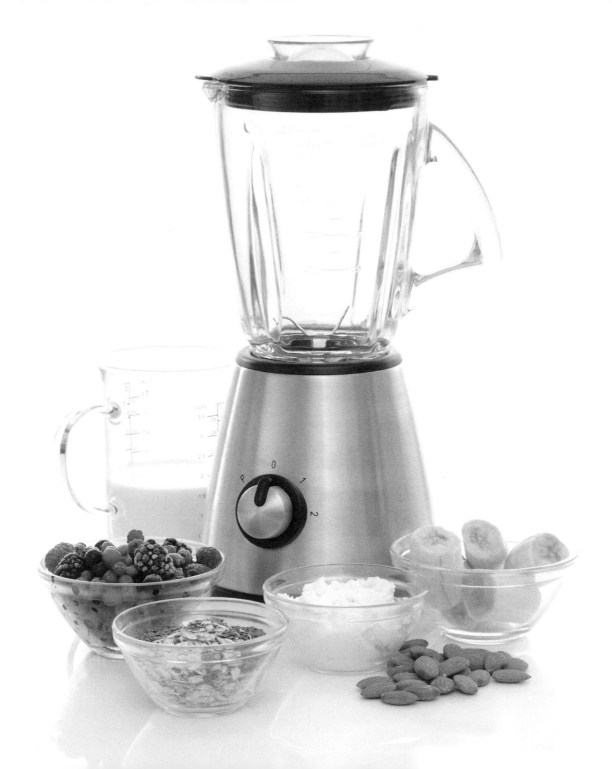

MAKE IT PRETTY

There is nothing wrong with a brown or gray smoothie except for the fact that it is not pretty, but who wants to eat or drink unappealing dishes? Being a painter and knowing how to mix colors comes in handy sometimes for a cook, too.

NICE COLOR COMBINATIONS:

Blue and green—blueberries with cucumbers, spinach, or other greens

Blue and red—blueberries with beets or strawberries

Orange and red—peaches or mangoes with strawberries or beets

Pineapple is pale yellow and can go with green, blue, or red.

Cucumbers are pale enough to work with red or orange colors without muting them too much.

UNAPPEALING COLOR COMBINATIONS:

Green and red—beets with spinach, green kale, etc.

Green and orange—carrots and spinach, kale, etc.

Blue and red with green—blueberries and strawberries with spinach or kale.

- Water, vegan milk, fruit juice, and mild or sweet vegetable juices such as celery, fennel, cucumber, and carrot juice work nicely as liquid in smoothies. I usually prefer unsweetened soy milk in smoothies because of the protein it has to offer. Hemp is the next highest in protein but homemade Basic Almond Milk (see page 40) is perhaps the most delicious.

- To freeze bananas for smoothies, simply peel them and place them in a ziplock bag in the freezer. **Don't forget to peel them!**

- If you don't have frozen bananas on hand, try throwing in a few ice cubes.

- Smoothies taste best when served immediately.

- Just about any type of nuts work for smoothies: Walnuts and pecans are perfect for smoothies, but cashews, macadamias, and pine nuts are the creamiest, so feel free to mix and match.

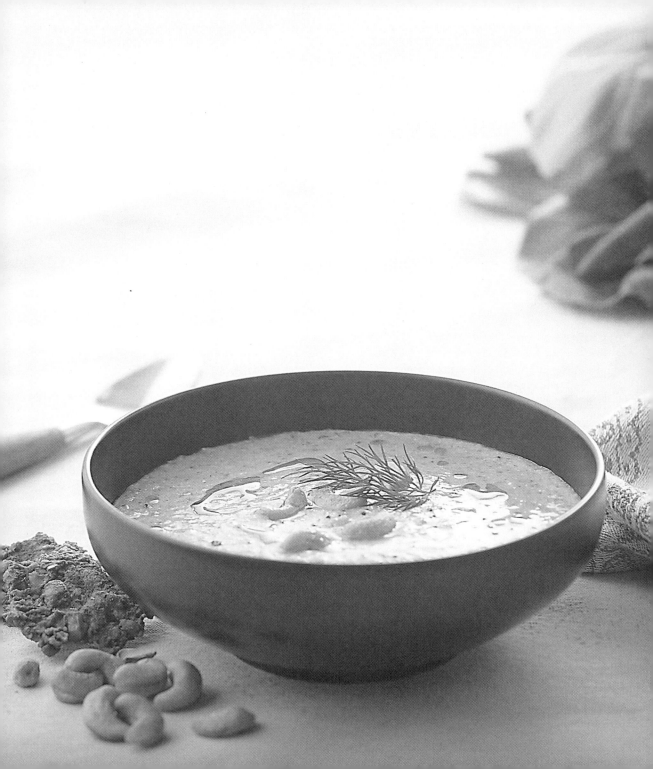

CHAPTER 4

SOUPS AND SALADS

Nuts in your soup? Yes, if you like delicious creamy soups without the saturated fat of dairy cream. The consistency that nuts can provide to a soup is truly exquisite! Any soup that is traditionally made with cream can be made with nut cream. See the recipes for Almond Cream (page 42) and Hazelnut Cream (page 44), and try them in the Hazelnut, Asparagus, and Mushroom Cream Soup (page 55) in this chapter. If you don't have nut milk or cream already made, try a handful of cashews or, better yet, pine nuts, blended right into the soup. Believe me, you will get compliments! The Cauliflower Cream Soup with Potatoes and Peas (page 54) is an example of the successful inclusion of nuts in soup and so is the deceptively simple Bok Choy Cream Soup (below). If you are not in the mood for a cream soup, try the Winter Squash Soup (page 56) with its pecan garnish.

BOK CHOY CREAM SOUP

MAKES ABOUT 6 SERVINGS

A few years back I had a job with a local organic farm creating recipes and providing samples of vegetables that were hard to sell. The sampled vegetables would go from being unpopular to selling out when people learned delicious and easy ways to use them! This soup was one of those recipes.

8 cups coarsely chopped bok choy (about 1½ pounds)

3 cups chopped onions (1 large)

3½ cups water

¾ cup cashews

¼ cup white miso or chickpea miso

½ teaspoon white pepper, or to taste

⅓ cup chopped fresh dill weed

1. Place the bok choy, onions, and water in a soup pot. Cover and bring to a boil. Reduce the heat to simmer and cook for about 10 minutes, or until the vegetables are tender.

2. Place the vegetables and their broth in a blender with the cashews and miso and blend until very smooth and creamy. Do this in batches, if necessary.

3. Return the soup to the pot and add the pepper. Mix well and either stir in the dill or use it as a garnish. Serve hot.

CAULIFLOWER CREAM SOUP WITH POTATOES AND PEAS

MAKES 6 TO 8 SERVINGS

No one will miss the cream in this delicate soup made creamy with pine nuts. Miso provides flavor and probiotics.

1 large cauliflower, cut into bite-size florets and pieces

4 medium potatoes, diced

1½ cups chopped onions

3 cups water

1 teaspoon herbs de Provence

2 cups unsweetened soy milk or other vegan milk

¼ cup white miso

½ cup pine nuts

½ teaspoon salt, if needed

½ teaspoon white pepper, or to taste

1 cup frozen peas

¼ cup finely chopped parsley, chives, or garlic chives

1. In a soup pot, combine the cauliflower, potatoes, onions, water, and herbs de Provence. Cover and bring to a boil. Reduce the heat and simmer for about 20 minutes, or until the vegetables are tender.

2. Transfer a portion of the soup to a blender. Add the milk, miso, pine nuts, salt (if needed), and white pepper. Blend until very smooth and creamy.

3. Return the blended mixture to the soup pot with the cooked ingredients and add the peas. Reheat if necessary, but do not boil.

4. Serve hot, garnished with parsley or chives.

NOTE: I like to blend part of this soup and leave some of it chunky, but if you prefer, you can blend it all to have a pureé. The proportions are up to you.

To protect the probiotic properties of the miso, when you reheat this soup, do so gently and do not bring it to a boil.

CELERY AND BASIL CREAM SOUP

MAKES 4 SERVINGS

If you have nuts in the freezer or fridge, you can always whip up something luxurious and delicious without having to run to the store. This quick and easy soup came about when there wasn't much on hand besides onions and celery and some basil in the garden. It would even be good with a teaspoon of dry basil, or another herb you like.

1 tablespoon olive oil

1½ cups chopped onions

3 cups chopped celery

1 cup fresh basil leaves

1 cup whole raw cashews

3 cups water

½ teaspoon salt

½ teaspoon white pepper

Minced parsley, chiffonade of basil, or garnish of choice

1. In a large pan, heat the olive oil. Add the onions and celery, cover, and sauté over medium-low for about 10 minutes, or until tender, stirring often.

2. Transfer about half the sautéed mixture to a blender. Add the basil, cashews, and 2 cups of the water. Blend until very smooth and creamy, then return it to the pan with the remaining onions and celery.

3. Add the rest of the water and the salt. Bring to a simmer while stirring. The soup should immediately thicken. Add the pepper. Mix well and serve topped with the garnish.

HAZELNUT, ASPARAGUS, AND MUSHROOM CREAM SOUP

MAKES 4 TO 6 SERVINGS

The hazelnuts in this soup provide a distinctive flavor that is delicious with the vegetables. Of course, you could substitute almond cream for the hazelnut cream for an equally good but different result.

2 tablespoons olive oil

1½ cups chopped onions

1 cup chopped celery

3 cups sliced mushrooms (8 ounces)

2 cups trimmed and sliced asparagus (12 ounces)

2 teaspoons herbs de Provence

¼ cup garbanzo flour

2 cups water

½ teaspoon salt, or to taste

2 cups Hazelnut Cream (page 44)

1. Heat the oil in a large, heavy pan. Add the onions and celery, cover, and sauté over medium heat, stirring often, for 5 to 10 minutes, or until the celery is tender.

2. Add the mushrooms and asparagus, stir, and cook for about 2 minutes.

3. Sprinkle the flour with one hand into the pan of vegetables while stirring constantly with the other hand.

4. When the flour is mixed in, slowly pour the water into the pan, while stirring vigorously. Bring to a boil and add the salt. Add the nut cream. Stir and serve.

PECAN-TOPPED WINTER SQUASH SOUP

MAKES 6 TO 8 SERVINGS

This savory soup, with slowly sautéed onions and garlic, is delicately spiced. The pecan topping makes it special and good enough for a holiday meal or any fall or winter occasion.

2 tablespoons olive oil

1 teaspoon whole fennel seed

1 teaspoon whole cumin seed

1 tablespoon fresh grated ginger

1½ cups chopped red onions

4 to 6 cloves garlic, minced

4½ cups mashed butternut squash

4 cups water

1 teaspoon salt

½ teaspoon ground fenugreek

½ teaspoon cinnamon

Cayenne to taste

1 cup chopped roasted pecans

1. Heat the oil in a large, heavy soup pot and add the fennel and cumin seeds. Cook over medium-high heat until the seeds pop, then add the ginger and onions. Mix well and add the garlic. Cover and reduce the heat to low.

2. Cook the onion mixture over low heat, stirring occasionally for 15–20 minutes, or until they are well done and starting to brown.

3. Add the squash, water, salt, fenugreek, and cinnamon. Whisk and bring to a simmer.

4. Taste for seasoning and add cayenne, if desired. Serve piping hot in bowls topped with chopped roasted pecans.

NOTE: For best flavor and sweetness, bake the squash rather than steaming it. To bake, either cut the squash in half and remove the seeds and stringy parts, or simply puncture it with a knife, and clean it out after it is baked. Place the squash on a baking sheet and bake at 350°F for 45 minutes, or until a knife can be easily inserted through the flesh, then scoop out the flesh with a spoon.

CREAMY PINE NUT GAZPACHO

MAKES 4 TO 6 SERVINGS

This is a scrumptious twist on a classic cold soup. Try it for a delicious, quick, and light lunch with a slice of whole-grain bread, and perhaps some hummus or other bean spread.

4 medium tomatoes, coarsely chopped

½ cup pine nuts

2 tablespoons red wine vinegar

½ teaspoon salt

1 medium cucumber, grated

1 scallion, chopped

¼ cup fresh chopped or chiffonade of basil

1. Place the tomatoes, pine nuts, vinegar, and salt in a blender, and puree until very smooth and creamy. Transfer to a bowl.

2. Add the cucumber and scallions to the bowl and stir. Top with the basil and serve immediately.

CLEAN OUT THE REFRIGERATOR SOUP

I often make a Clean Out the Refrigerator Soup with little odds and ends of vegetables that would otherwise go to waste. There is no recipe because just about anything can be used as long as it is fresh enough to be healthy and tasty.

Simply put vegetables and water together in a large pan. If you are not used to improvising, use less water than you might think you will need, because vegetables contain their own water. More water can be added as the soup cooks, if needed, because it is easier to add more water than to fix a soup that is too watery.

Cover the pan and bring the soup to a boil. Then reduce the heat and simmer until the vegetables are tender. Place some or all of the cooked vegetables in a blender with a handful of pine nuts, blanched almonds, or cashews and blend until very creamy. (If you like your creamy soup with some pieces in it, only blend about half the vegetables.) Add herbs near the end of cooking and add either some salt or white or yellow miso to taste.

The trick is to blend it very well so that there is no a gritty texture. The nuts can be soaked first, or not. Either way will be delicious. Just remember that cashews will add a slight sweetness to the soup, so if that isn't what you want, use pine nuts or blanched almonds. Start with a handful; and if more richness is desired, add some more.

Instead of buying broth for soups, I just use water (no one has ever accused me of having flavorless soups) along with some of the water from cooking the vegetables. Leftover cooking water can be kept in the freezer either as ice cubes or a frozen block and added to the pot with the other ingredients for future soups.

- Zucchini and other summer squash with onions. This simple soup, prepared with herbs and spices to taste, is surprisingly good.

- Green beans, onions, and potatoes. One year I had so many green beans in the garden that I froze a lot of them. Blended into a simple soup like this, frozen green beans are fabulous!

- Potatoes, carrots, yellow squash, celery, onions, and corn. Blend about half of these ingredients with nuts, and leave the rest chunky for a creamy chowder.

- Potatoes, onions, and broccoli or a leafy vegetable such as collards, kale, mustard, or turnip greens. This is a delicious, easy, and satisfying way to get the nutritional benefits from these dark green vegetables.

USING MISO

Miso adds flavor and healthful probiotics to soups, sauces, salad dressings, and dips. Always remember to add it after the dish is cooked, in order not to kill the beneficial bacteria in the miso. If you reheat a soup or other dish containing miso, don't bring it to a boil. Warm it up until it is pleasantly hot, but don't cook it.

KEEP IT PRETTY

This is just for looks. The soup's presentation doesn't affect its taste; but as any painter knows, orange and green make brown, and a brown soup or smoothie is not very pretty. The French say, "We eat first with our eyes."

So keep your colors clean and blend together vegetables that are in the same color range. For instance, if a soup is going to be blended, don't add a red bell pepper, beets, carrots, or winter squash to lots of greens. The same goes with smoothies. See page 51.

GARNISHES FOR SOUPS

A garnish can make a big difference in how a soup tastes and looks. It adds eye appeal, but when nuts are used as the garnish, they add interesting texture, too. Other good garnishes for soups include chopped herbs. Try the savory Walnut and Shallot Bread (page 99), toasted and cut into little squares and floated on top of a soup for something really good.

SALADS

Nuts in salads are a pretty common sight, but here in *Superfood Nuts*, it was my goal to bring you some salads using vegetables that you might not know what to do with, such as kohlrabi, jicama, and Belgian endive, and to provide a different twist on more common vegetables such as beets, because it is always fun to try something new. Also, did you know that it helps your local farmers when you buy some of the lesser-known vegetables that they grow? That's because these are often vegetables that grow particularly well and need less attention to produce prolifically than some of the more familiar ones.

When adding nuts to salads, don't forget that these recipes offer only a fraction of what you can do. Just a handful adds nutrition, satisfaction, richness, and texture to almost any type of salad, and it's almost impossible to go wrong. A garnish of walnuts or pecans can elevate a simple green salad from ordinary to wow! So please try these recipes, and then go ahead and create your own. Don't forget that in the Sauces, Gravies, Dressings, and Whips section of this book there are several delicious salad dressings made mostly from nuts!

BARLEY WALNUT SALAD

MAKES ABOUT 4 SERVINGS

There is something about the combination of barley and walnuts that is really delicious. We tend to think of barley as a hearty grain to use in a winter soup, but in traditional Chinese medicine it is considered cooling and in this easy salad it is quite refreshing.

2 cups cooked barley

1 cup halved grapes

¾ cup chopped celery

¾ cup chopped walnuts

½ cup minced parsley

2 tablespoons balsamic vinegar

1 tablespoon Dijon-style mustard

1 teaspoon dried tarragon

½ teaspoon salt

Freshly ground black pepper

1. In a large bowl, combine the barley, grapes, celery, walnuts, and parsley.

2. In a small bowl, stir together the vinegar and mustard. Add the tarragon and salt. Mix well and add to the salad. Toss and add the pepper to taste and serve, or refrigerate and serve later.

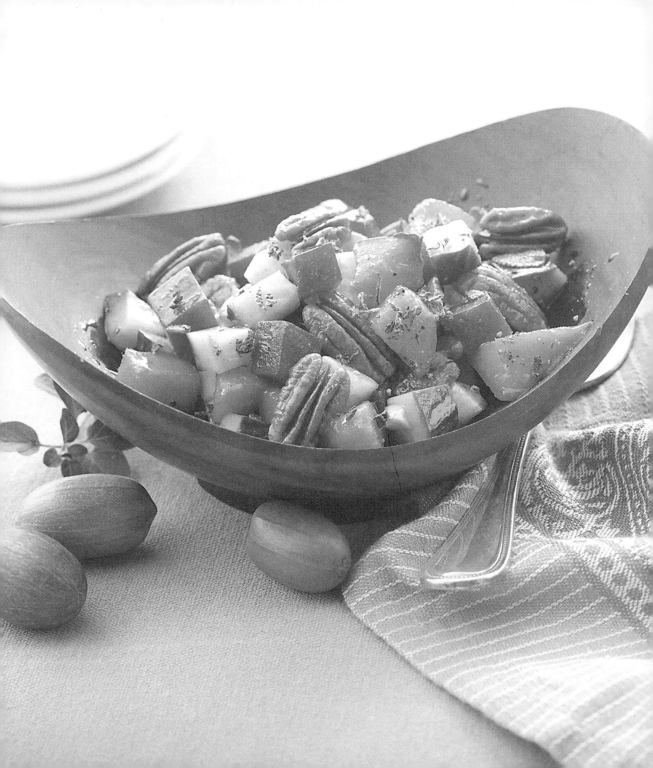

BEET AND PECAN SALAD WITH MANGO AND CUCUMBER

MAKES ABOUT 6 SERVINGS

I have always been fond of beets with oranges, but when I wanted to test this recipe with oranges there were no oranges to be found. However, there were plenty of mangoes in my backyard. Everybody loved it this way—it could be made with either mangoes or oranges and still be delish! We had it as a side dish for dinner, then the next day I mixed it with leftover quinoa for a wonderful lunch.

4 cups diced beets (4 medium)

1½ cups diced cucumbers (1 large)

1½ cups diced mangoes (1 large)

1 cup pecans

2 cloves garlic, pressed

¼ cup fresh minced sage

2 tablespoons orange-infused olive oil

2 tablespoons tamari

2 tablespoons balsamic vinegar

1. Steam or pressure-cook the beets in a small amount of water until they are tender. Drain, if necessary and transfer to a salad bowl to cool. Steaming should take 20–30 minutes; for pressure cooking, they just need to be brought to pressure.

2. When the beets have cooled to at least room temperature, add the remaining ingredients. Mix and serve immediately, or chill and serve later.

NOTE: Orange-infused olive oil can be purchased in stores that sell imported Italian oils and vinegars. As a substitute, about 1 tablespoon grated orange zest can be added to regular good-quality olive oil.

CABBAGE SALAD WITH WALNUTS AND RAISINS

MAKES 4 TO 6 SERVINGS

This recipe started out as something totally different. At the time, my taste buds were set on tarragon, which I didn't have, but lemon zest, ginger, and garlic made a delightful alternative. It is a great recipe to take to a potluck because it is easy to make and holds up well. The walnuts in this salad can be either raw or roasted.

4 cups shredded cabbage

1 cup shredded carrots

1 cup walnuts, in halves or chopped

¼ cup raisins

3 tablespoons lemon juice

2 tablespoons walnut oil or flaxseed oil

1 tablespoon grated lemon zest

1 tablespoon grated ginger

1 clove garlic, pressed

½ teaspoon salt

1. Combine all the ingredients in a salad bowl.

2. Mix and serve immediately, or chill and serve later.

TIP: Both walnut oil and flaxseed oil are prone to rancidity, so if you use one of these oils make sure it is fresh. Olive oil can be substituted.

CHOPPED SALAD WITH WALNUTS

MAKES ABOUT 6 SERVINGS

This salad is colorful and delicious with a simple meal of lentils and rice but would be good with just about anything.

3 cups chopped radicchio (1 medium head)

2 cups chopped Belgian endive (3 small heads)

1 cup diced cucumbers (½ medium)

¼ cup chopped scallions

½ cup thinly sliced radishes

½ cup thinly sliced fennel (½ small bulb)

1 cup cherry tomatoes, halved

1 cup walnut halves

DRESSING

2 tablespoons tamari

2 tablespoons balsamic vinegar

2 tablespoons olive oil

1 tablespoon prepared mustard

1 clove garlic, pressed

1 teaspoon tarragon

1. In a salad bowl, combine the vegetables and walnuts.

2. In a small jar or bowl, combine the dressing ingredients. Shake or stir.

3. Add about half the dressing to the salad and taste it. If you want more, add the rest. If not, save it for something else.

NOTE: The variety of tomatoes I used for this salad were Sungold, which are sweet and low acid. They made a delicious addition to the slightly bitter endive and radicchio, but any small sweet tomato will work.

The mustard I used in this particular dressing was organic yellow mustard. For years, I had only used Dijon-style mustard, considering yellow mustard sort of a junk food. But this one had only quality ingredients, and the yellow is from turmeric, which provides a delicious flavor variation.

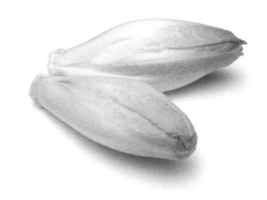

JICAMA, ORANGE, AND PISTACHIO SALAD

MAKES 4 TO 6 SERVINGS

Jicama is a very low-calorie and high-fiber root vegetable. It is an excellent source of oligofructose inulin, which is said to stimulate the growth of beneficial intestinal bacteria. This is my new favorite salad, because it is refreshing and exotic with a hint of spice. It is also so good that it needs neither salt nor oil to be delicious!

4 cups grated jicama

2 cups sliced orange segments

½ cup lightly roasted pistachios

2 tablespoons lime juice

1 tablespoon grated orange zest

1 teaspoon cumin

¼ teaspoon ground chipotle

1. Combine all ingredients in a salad bowl.

2. Mix well and serve. Leftovers can be stored overnight in the refrigerator in a covered container and are just as delicious the next day. This recipe is good stored for 3–4 days, but is probably best if you don't keep it too long.

KAMUT, GREEN BEAN, AND NUT SALAD

MAKES 4 TO 6 SERVINGS

This is good at any time of year, but it makes a beautiful dish for a Thanksgiving dinner. Everyone seems to like it and it holds up well. I have made it with walnuts, pecans, and hazelnuts, and they are all equally delicious, so it's your choice for this one!

1 cup kamut, soaked overnight and drained

3 cups water

1 pound green beans, about 3 cups trimmed and cut into 2-inch pieces

1 teaspoon dried sage

2 tablespoons olive oil

2 tablespoons balsamic vinegar

2 tablespoons tamari

2 tablespoons grated shallots

1 tablespoon Dijon-style mustard

1 cup freshly roasted, unsalted nuts

1. Place the kamut in a pan with the water. Cover, bring to a boil, reduce the heat, and simmer for 30 to 40 minutes, or until tender. Drain off any excess water and transfer to a mixing bowl.

2. Cook the green beans until tender-crisp, and transfer them to the bowl with the cooked grain.

3. Add the sage, olive oil, balsamic vinegar, tamari, shallots, and mustard. Either mix well with the kamut and beans and serve immediately or chill for later. Add the nuts just before serving, either on top of the salad or mixed in.

NOTE: To turn this salad into a satisfying meal, I sauté some prebaked and seasoned tofu and serve it along with the Kamut, Green Bean, and Nut Salad atop a bed of greens.

TIP—GREEN BEANS AU POINT

One of my pet peeves is green beans that are over- or undercooked. Because most everyone's grandma had, at one time or another, overcooked green beans, the pendulum swung in the other direction and it became fashionable to undercook them. One is not better than the other, because to be truly delicious they need to be done just right. I can't give you a time for this because it depends on the beans themselves, the pan you use, and the intensity of the heat. Of course, this is a matter of taste, but I think the French get it right in the small villages and country restaurants where they serve green beans that are pleasantly tender but still bright and somewhat firm.

My favorite way to cook green beans is in a pressure cooker. I bring them to pressure and then cool the pressure cooker down quickly under running water and open it immediately. They will be perfect 99 percent of the time. If you steam them instead, just pick one out every so often and test it for doneness. Look at your food, not your watch, when cooking.

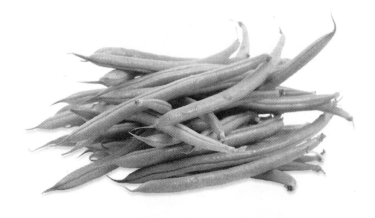

KOHLRABI PECAN SALAD

MAKES 6 SERVINGS

Ever wonder what to do with a kohlrabi bulb? Take this recipe to a potluck, and most people won't have a clue what they are eating; but they will eat it anyway because it's good! This salad stores well and is just as good, or better, the next day.

1 teaspoon olive oil

1 tablespoon fennel seeds

3 cups peeled and diced kohlrabi bulb, leaves removed (1 large)

2 cups diced Pink Lady apples (2 medium)

1 tablespoon lemon juice

1 or 2 tablespoons balsamic vinegar, to taste

2 tablespoons olive oil

½ cup pecan halves

⅓ cup parsley

Freshly ground black pepper, to taste

1. In a small saucepan, heat the olive oil. Add the fennel seeds and stir them until they begin to pop. Set aside.

2. In a mixing bowl, combine the kohlrabi, apples, and lemon juice. Mix well.

3. Add the vinegar, oil, pecans, parsley, and roasted fennel seeds. Add the pepper, toss, and serve.

NOTE: Did you know that kohlrabi leaves are delicious cooked like collard greens? They are slightly sweeter and perhaps even more tender than collards, and can be steamed, pressure cooked, or added to soups and stews.

LENTIL WALNUT SALAD WITH BELGIAN ENDIVE

MAKES 4 TO 6 SERVINGS

This is really good, but if you splurge on some high-quality balsamic vinegar it is even better.

1 cup small, whole green lentils

3 cups water

5 bay leaves

1 teaspoon fennel seeds

2 tablespoons olive oil

2 tablespoons balsamic vinegar

1 tablespoon tamari

1 teaspoon herbs de Provence

2 cups Belgian endive, coarsely chopped (about 3 small heads)

¼ cup finely chopped parsley, chives, or garlic chives

¾ cup chopped walnuts (roasted or raw)

1. Sort and rinse the lentils. Look for stones and discolored, moldy, or broken beans, and discard any you find. Place them in a medium-size saucepan with the water, bay leaves, and fennel seeds. Cover and bring to a boil. Reduce the heat and simmer for about 40 minutes, or until the water is absorbed. Transfer the hot, cooked lentils to a mixing bowl.

2. Add the olive oil, vinegar, tamari, and herbs de Provence. Let cool.

3. Add the endive, and either mix or garnish with the parsley or chives. Serve on a bed of salad greens. The walnuts can either be mixed into the salad or served on top of it.

MY FAVORITE DRESSING

I have made this dressing for years, and it takes only a couple of minutes. Store it in the refrigerator and serve it over any salad or steamed vegetable. Try it over a plain salad of garden-fresh greens and top it with a handful of nuts and you are sure to get compliments!

1 part tamari
1 part balsamic vinegar
2 parts olive oil

Mix together the ingredients in a jar and add the following flavor variations to taste: Pressed garlic, prepared mustard, tarragon, or other fresh herbs.

FRUIT SALAD BLISS

A fruit salad is delicious with a handful of just about any type of nuts, but if you want something amazing, try the Peaches and Pine Nut Cream (page 75) or the Walnut Apricot Breakfast Whip (page 75) to dress a fruit salad—it is divine!

KEEPING NUTS CRISP
IN THE SALAD

To keep nuts crisp until they are added to a salad, add them last, and if you are planning to keep the salad a couple of days, store the nuts in a small bag or container separate from the salad. If you don't want to bother, it is no big deal, but the nuts will not be as crisp.

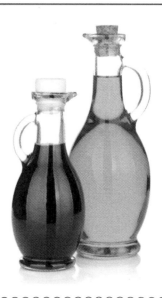

TIP—NUTTY VARIATIONS ON CARROT SALAD

A grated carrot salad is an easy addition to a meal, especially when the other vegetables in the meal are green, because it offers a great color contrast. Adding nuts always makes this ordinary salad a lot more interesting.

Here are some variation ideas for a carrot salad:

• Chopped raw walnuts with lemon juice, a bit of grated lemon zest, tarragon, and olive oil.

• Chopped pecans, raisins, and balsamic vinegar with minced tangerine peel.

• Pistachios, grated orange peel, cumin, lemon.

• Toasted almonds, thinly sliced dried apricots.

• Grated jicama, chopped macadamia nuts, lime juice, and chipotle.

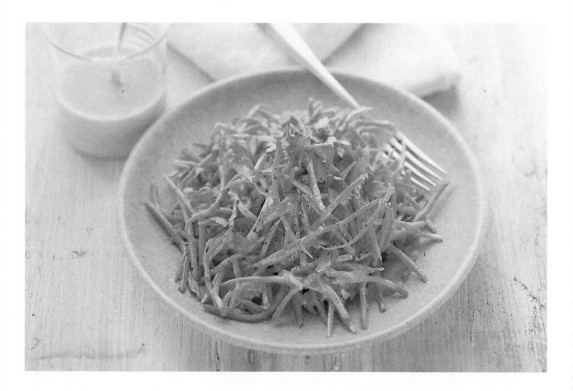

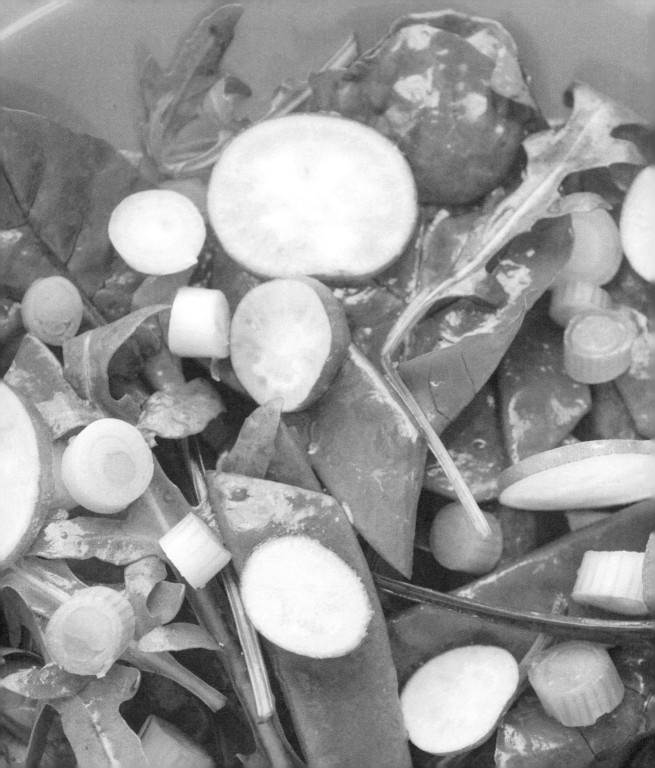

CHAPTER 5

SAUCES, GRAVIES, DRESSINGS, AND WHIPS

Do you buy your salad dressings? Are you confident enough to quickly whip up a sauce or gravy? If you answered "no" to either of these questions, you are in for a treat! These dressing recipes are as easy to make as a smoothie, and everyone will ask what makes them so delicious. The answer is nuts! Yes, nuts furnish all the fat in these creamy dressings, so there is no need for extracted oils, and nuts are so nutritious that you can enjoy these dressings in moderation, of course, knowing you are eating something that is good for you. Doesn't it stand to reason that the dressing you pour on your salad should be as fresh as the salad itself? So many bottled dressings contain ingredients such as sugar, cheap and highly refined oils, and additives. When you see how easy and delicious these healthy, homemade dressings are, the bottled dressings will totally lose their appeal. The Creamy Pine Nut Dressing (page 72) is so mild and yummy that even I was surprised the first time I tasted it! Each of these dressings relies on a different nut and different seasonings to go with it, so make sure to try them all to discover your favorites. Just remember that, unlike most conventional dressings, these contain water, so use them up within a week while they are fresh. I don't think this will be difficult to do, though.

Another thing to know about these dressings is that they are not intended exclusively for salads. They are equally good over steamed vegetables, baked potatoes, and cooked grain dishes! For example, I served the Pistachio Dressing (page 73) with cumin and quinoa topped with steamed vegetables. There was a salad on the side, on the same plate and with the same dressing. This was a quick weekday meal and the ingredients were fresh, so it was good and easy.

The fruit and nut whips are also wonderful. I considered putting them in the Breakfast chapter, because that is when I usually use them, or the Dessert chapter, because they would be equally good over cake or pie. But they ended up in Sauces, Gravies, and Dressings because that's what they actually are. But feel free to try them with lots of different dishes, from fruit salad and pancakes to dessert. They can be made sweeter with the addition of dates, coconut nectar, or even a few drops of stevia. You can also experiment with the type of nuts and fruits used. It's pretty hard to go wrong with such simple and delicious ingredients.

Nuts also add a delicious rich creaminess and flavor to gravies and sauces. The Cashew Béchamel Sauce on this page is as good as any traditional béchamel, and is dairy free. The Pecan Sage Gravy (facing page) over mashed potatoes will fill the nostalgia void whenever you want some down-home comfort food that is healthy at the same time! Did you know that nut butter, or nuts blended with liquid as is the case with these recipes, will thicken a sauce when it's cooked as if you added flour? This is quite convenient for making sauces and gravies, but unlike sauces made with flour, these do not have the tendency to lump.

SAVORY SAUCES AND GRAVY

CASHEW BÉCHAMEL SAUCE

MAKES ABOUT 2 CUPS

This is as rich and creamy as any béchamel you have tasted. It is also mild enough to deliciously complement anything you choose to serve it with. Try it over asparagus or broccoli, with spinach, etc. For an old-fashioned luncheon, try it with carrots, peas, and mushrooms over toast for a taste of midcentury elegance! The trick to this recipe is to make sure the nuts are blended until totally smooth.

1 cup cashews
2 cups water
½ teaspoon salt
¼ teaspoon freshly grated nutmeg
¼ teaspoon white pepper

1. Place the cashews, water, and salt in a blender and blend 2 to 3 minutes or until very smooth and creamy, taking as long as needed.

2. Transfer the mixture to a medium-size saucepan and whisk over medium heat until the sauce comes to a simmer. It will thicken immediately.

3. Remove the pan from the heat and stir in the nutmeg and pepper.

4. The sauce will thicken upon setting, so add more water if necessary.

PECAN SAGE GRAVY

MAKES 1½ CUPS

Enjoy the flavors of the holidays anytime with this delicious gravy. You can serve it over mashed potatoes, quinoa, tempeh, or any other food that could use a rich and flavorful gravy.

1 cup pecans

1½ cups water

1 tablespoon plus 1 teaspoon tamari

1 teaspoon dried sage (or 2 tablespoons fresh)

½ teaspoon white pepper

1. Coarsely grind the pecans in a blender.

2. Transfer the ground pecans to a skillet and stir over medium-high heat until they become fragrant, then transfer them back to the blender.

3. Add the water, tamari, sage, and white pepper. Blend until very smooth.

4. Transfer the blended mixture back to the skillet and stir over medium-high heat until the gravy begins to simmer. While stirring constantly, continue cooking for 2 to 3 minutes, or until it thickens.

WALNUT SAUCE

MAKES 1½ CUPS

Use this savory sauce over vegetables or grain dishes. It is great on asparagus, broccoli, or just about any vegetable.

1½ cups water or unseasoned vegetable stock

1 cup walnut halves

⅓ cup nutritional yeast

1 teaspoon turmeric powder

1 clove garlic

½ teaspoon salt

1. Place all ingredients in a blender and blend 1 to 2 minutes or until smooth and creamy.

2. Transfer mixture to a saucepan and cook over medium heat until it is thickened to the desired consistency.

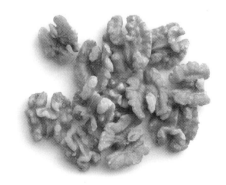

DRESSINGS

CREAMY PINE NUT DRESSING

MAKES ABOUT 1 CUP

This dressing is pure deliciousness as far as I'm concerned! Pine nuts make up for the lack of extracted oil in this delicately flavored but savory dressing.

½ cup pine nuts

½ cup water

2 tablespoons white wine vinegar

1 tablespoon Dijon-style mustard

1 clove garlic

¼ teaspoon salt

1. Place all the ingredients in a blender and blend until very smooth and creamy.

2. Use immediately or transfer to a jar with a lid and store in the refrigerator for up to a week.

PECAN DRESSING

MAKES ABOUT 1¼ CUPS

The pecans provide flavor and creaminess, nutritional yeast makes it rich in B vitamins, and the garlic and thyme make a dressing that is delicious any way you serve it. Try it on cooked greens as well as raw salads.

½ cup pecan halves

½ cup water

½ cup nutritional yeast

2 tablespoons cider vinegar

2 cloves garlic

½ to ¾ teaspoon salt, to taste

½ teaspoon thyme

Freshly ground black pepper, to taste

1. Place all the ingredients in a blender, and blend until very smooth and creamy.

2. Use immediately or transfer to a jar with a lid and store in the refrigerator for up to a week.

MUSHROOM PESTO

MAKES ABOUT 1¼ CUPS

I wanted to do something that tasted somewhat like a traditional pesto, but with more nuts, a little less oil, and of course is vegan, so the idea of adding sautéed mushrooms to provide flavor and body along with the nutritional yeast, which gives a cheesy flavor, worked beautifully. If by any chance you have some truffle salt, add it to this pesto instead of plain salt for even more flavor.

1 tablespoon olive oil

1½ cups sliced mushrooms

2 cups fresh basil leaves, lightly packed

3 cloves garlic

⅓ cup olive oil

1 cup walnuts

¼ cup nutritional yeast

½ teaspoon salt

1. Heat the olive oil in a skillet. Add the mushrooms and sauté for 3 to 5 minutes, or until heated through and tender. Let cool to room temperature.

2. Place the basil leaves and garlic in a blender or food processor and start to grind over low speed. Drizzle in the olive oil, and then stop the machine, add the sautéed mushrooms, walnuts, yeast, and salt.

3. Grind until everything is mixed but not completely smooth. Use a rubber spatula to scrape the sides of the machine, if needed. Serve with pasta, potatoes, or quinoa.

PISTACHIO DRESSING

MAKES ABOUT 1 CUP

You may be surprised by the fresh, light taste provided by the lime in this simple dressing. Who says a recipe needs a long list of ingredients to be good? This is delicious with all sorts of vegetables, cooked and raw.

½ cup roasted, unsalted pistachios

⅓ cup water

¼ cup chopped sweet onions

¼ teaspoon salt, to taste

¼ cup lime juice

1. Place all the ingredients in a blender, and blend 1 to 2 minutes or until very smooth and creamy.

2. Use immediately or transfer to a jar with a lid and store in the refrigerator for up to a week.

NOTE: This recipe is also good with ½ teaspoon cumin added to the blender with the other ingredients. Try the recipe without cumin first, but to serve with certain foods— such as corn on the cob without butter—the cumin adds a delicious twist.

TOMATO PINE NUT SAUCE

MAKES ABOUT 1 CUP

Use this delicious sauce as a salad dressing over steamed vegetables. It is especially good over baked potatoes or pasta. Use fresh local tomatoes at their peak of ripeness for the best results, but don't worry: Even with mediocre tomatoes, it is quite delicious!

1½ cups coarsely chopped tomatoes (1 large or 2 small)

½ cup pine nuts

1 to 2 cloves garlic

2 to 3 tablespoons lemon juice, to taste

1 teaspoon basil

1 tablespoon white or yellow miso, or more to taste

1. Blend together all ingredients in a blender until smooth and creamy.

2. Use immediately or transfer to a jar with a lid and store in the refrigerator for up to a week.

WALNUT DRESSING

MAKES ABOUT ¾ CUP

Creamy walnuts with fresh rosemary combine beautifully in this dressing. As with all these nut dressings, don't save them for just salads. Get creative and try them on all sorts of dishes, from grains to vegetables, as a healthful and delicious seasoning.

¾ cup walnut halves

½ cup water

1 tablespoon tamari

1 tablespoon balsamic vinegar

1 tablespoon chopped fresh rosemary

1. Place all the ingredients in a blender, and blend until very smooth and creamy.

2. Use immediately or transfer to a jar with a lid and store in the refrigerator for up to a week.

FRUIT AND NUT WHIPS

Breakfast or dessert, breakfast or dessert? I wasn't sure which chapter to put these scrumptious creams in because they could go in either one. A big dollop of either of these sauces for breakfast over a diced, perfectly ripe mango tastes almost too good to not be sinful. It would be equally delicious over cake, pie, or other dessert as a whipped topping. For dessert, however, you may want to add a few drops of stevia or a tablespoon of some other sweetener.

PEACHES AND PINE NUT CREAM

MAKES ABOUT 1 CUP

½ cup pine nuts

1 large ripe peach, in large chunks

1 teaspoon vanilla extract

1. Soak the pine nuts for 1 or 2 hours in water to cover.

2. Drain and discard the water.

3. Transfer the nuts to a blender, add the peach and vanilla, and blend 1 minute or until very smooth and creamy. Store in a covered container in the refrigerator for up to 4 days.

WALNUT APRICOT BREAKFAST WHIP

MAKES ABOUT 1½ CUPS

½ cup walnut halves

½ cup dried apricots

1 hot (not boiling) cup water

1 teaspoon vanilla extract

1. Place the walnuts and apricots in a medium-size bowl. Add the hot water and soak for about 30 minutes.

2. Place the soaked mixture, along with the soaking water, in a blender. Add the vanilla and blend until very creamy. Store in a covered container in the refrigerator for up to 4 days.

NOTE: Instead of heating the water, you can simply soak the fruit and nuts in room temperature water until the fruit is plumped.

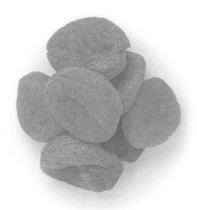

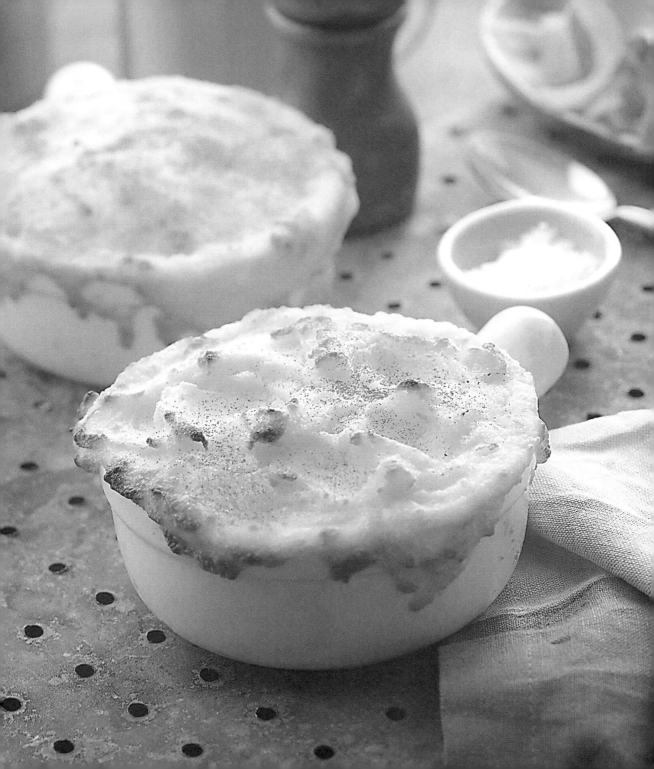

CHAPTER 6

MAIN DISHES

Nuts for dinner? Unless you are familiar with vegan or vegetarian cooking, you may be surprised by the variety of dishes that so beautifully lend themselves to the addition of nuts. Nuts are often thought of as a snack food or are limited to baked goods and desserts, but as you will discover in this chapter, they add a meaty and satisfying quality to any number of delicious main dishes.

You don't have to be a vegan or even aspire to be a vegan to enjoy these dishes. They are just plain good; and even if you have absolutely no interest in going vegan, you are likely to enjoy the occasional meatless meal using these recipes. There are serving suggestions with the main dish recipes in this chapter to help you to round out your menu so you can go meatless, whenever you like, without feeling that something is missing.

Nuts are often featured in holiday dishes. This tradition probably came about because the nuts we associate with the holidays—walnuts and pecans—are harvested in the fall, and are at their peak of freshness during late November and December. For a delicious holiday main dish, try the Holiday Pecan Tofu Loaf (page 83). Once I made this recipe for a vegetarian friend to take to a family Thanksgiving dinner, and he told me that

there were no leftovers because everyone wanted to try it, and once they tried it they wanted more! But he said there was plenty of leftover turkey. The Lentil Pie (page 85) also makes a fabulous holiday main dish. The Tempeh Walnut Shepherd's Pie (page 88) is a more simple-and-homey dish; but because it makes a lot of servings and is so popular, even it would make a good holiday dish. For an intimate fall or winter dinner, try the Quinoa-Stuffed Acorn Squash with Pecans (page 86). But don't get the wrong idea and wait for a holiday to enjoy these recipes. Except perhaps for the stuffed tofu loaf, they are all super easy to make and can be enjoyed any time of year.

For a sophisticated summer meal, try the Walnut-Topped Braised Mushrooms and Market Vegetables (page 90) over whole-grain pasta or quinoa. It is light and filling at the same time. The Eggplant with

Caramelized Onions, Walnuts, and Peas (page 82) is another easy one that is pretty sure to please. It is my goal to give vegans and vegetarians some great new options, while hopefully showing non-vegans that a meatless meal can hold its own and be favorably compared to anything out there in taste, texture, and appearance.

ALMOND CREAM SPINACH AND MUSHROOMS

MAKES 3 TO 4 SERVINGS

This is really good, especially over whole-wheat pasta! If you have the Almond Cream already made and a couple of bags of prewashed spinach on hand, dinner can be on the table in about 15 minutes! If you have some leftover pasta, it is even quicker. It is also good over quinoa.

1 tablespoon olive oil

1½ cups chopped onions

2 cups sliced mushrooms

10 ounces baby spinach

1 teaspoon savory (see Note)

2 tablespoons garbanzo flour

1 cup Almond Cream (see recipe page 42)

1 teaspoon salt, or less to taste

½ teaspoon white pepper, or less to taste

¼ teaspoon ground or freshly grated nutmeg

1. Heat the olive oil in a large, heavy pan. Add the onions and sauté over medium heat for 3 to 4 minutes, or until they are almost translucent. Add the mushrooms, spinach, and savory. If all the spinach does not fit into the pan, stir it over high heat for a minute to wilt just enough to make room for the rest. Cover and cook for 2 to 3 minutes, or until the spinach and mushrooms are done.

2. Place the garbanzo flour in one hand and sprinkle it into the pan with the cooked spinach mixture while stirring with the other hand. Stir until the flour is mixed in.

3. Slowly pour the Almond Cream into the pan with the vegetables while continuing to stir. Bring the mixture to a boil and add the salt, pepper, and nutmeg.

NOTE: This recipe is very versatile. Fresh dill weed or tarragon are delicious substitutes for the savory, and frozen peas would make a wonderful addition. In fact, this recipe can be made with just about any type of vegetable you may have on hand. Broccoli, asparagus, carrots, and summer squash would all be good additions to, or substitutions for, the spinach and mushrooms.

BARLEY AND OYSTER MUSHROOMS WITH VEGETABLES AND WALNUTS

MAKES 4 GENEROUS SERVINGS

Barley is an old-fashioned grain that too often gets passed by for either trendier or more common ones. It has a delicious light and chewy texture and is marvelous with nuts. With a salad that contains some beans or tofu, this recipe makes a meal.

1 cup pearled barley

3 cups water

2 large stalks broccoli, stems included (one bunch)

10 ounces baby spinach (about 4 cups)

10 ounces oyster mushrooms (about 4 cups)

1 tablespoon olive oil

1½ cups chopped onions

3 tablespoons tamari

2 tablespoons mirin or white wine

1 tablespoon white wine vinegar, rice vinegar, or cider vinegar

2 teaspoons herbs de Provence

1 cup walnut halves, raw or roasted, as desired

1. Rinse the barley and place it in a medium-size pan with the water. Cover, bring to a boil, then reduce the heat and simmer for about 45 minutes, or until the barley is tender and the water is absorbed.

2. While the barley is cooking, prep the veggies. Peel and chop the broccoli stems, and separate the florets into bite-size pieces. Wash the spinach, if necessary, and trim the mushrooms, slicing off the tough parts on the bottoms.

3. Heat the olive oil in a large skillet. Add the onions and broccoli stems and sauté over medium-high heat until the onions are translucent. Add the broccoli florets, tamari, mirin, and vinegar. Stir, cover, and cook for 3 to 4 minutes, or until the broccoli starts to get tender, stirring often.

4. Add the spinach, mushrooms, and herbs de Provence. Stir and cover for a minute. Then remove the lid and sauté until the mushrooms are cooked.

5. To serve, either add the barley to the vegetables and mix, or serve the vegetables over the barley. Top with walnuts and serve immediately.

TIP: This recipe can be easily varied to use any type of vegetable or mushroom that you have on hand.

BARLEY WALNUT BURGERS

*MAKES 8 BURGERS
(APPROXIMATELY 3 INCHES IN
DIAMETER AND ¾ INCH THICK)*

These are good either plain or with a sauce. Since they are grain burgers, they are best served on a plate with vegetables and not on a bun. Try them with a tomato or light mushroom sauce for a real treat.

1 cup pearled barley

3½ cups water

½ cup nutritional yeast

¾ cup coarsely ground walnuts

¼ cup minced parsley

¼ cup minced celery

2 cloves garlic, pressed

1 teaspoon dried sage

½ teaspoon dried thyme

1 teaspoon salt

½ teaspoon white pepper

2 tablespoons olive oil, as needed

1. In a medium-size pan, combine the barley and water. Cover, bring to a boil, then reduce the heat and simmer for about 45 minutes, or until the barley is tender and the water is absorbed. Let it cool for at least 10 minutes before proceeding.

2. Add the yeast, walnuts, parsley, celery, garlic, sage, thyme, and salt. Mix well and form into 8 patties, pressing firmly between your hands. If the mixture is too hot to comfortably handle, wait a few more minutes.

3. Heat the olive oil in a skillet and cook the burgers for 4 to 5 minutes, or until each is toasty brown on the bottom. Turn them over and brown the other side.

NOTE: The patties can be made in advance and stored in the refrigerator until dinner time, then browned just before serving. This recipe uses 3½ cups water rather than the usual 3 cups because the little bit of extra water makes the grain a bit stickier and helps the burgers hold together.

CRUSTLESS SPINACH WALNUT PIE

MAKES 4 SERVINGS

This dish reminds me of a vegan version of the Persian dish KooKoo. You may be amazed at how much spinach you can eat when it is prepared like this! It is delicious with a carrot salad and a grain dish or some roasted potatoes.

16 ounces fresh spinach

1 teaspoon salt, divided

¼ cup dehydrated shallots or onions

12.3-ounce package firm silken tofu

¾ cup ground walnuts

1 teaspoon dried thyme

1 teaspoon turmeric

½ teaspoon white pepper

¼ cup chopped walnuts

1. Preheat the oven to 350°F. Oil and flour an 8 × 8-inch square baking dish.

2. Place the spinach and ½ teaspoon salt in a large pan. Cover and cook until the spinach is wilted. Transfer the spinach to a colander to drain, and press out some of the excess liquid using a spatula. Place the spinach in a mixing bowl. Add the shallots or onions.

3. Coarsely grind the walnuts in a blender.

4. Place the tofu with the remaining ½ teaspoon salt in a blender and blend until it is smooth. Add to the mixing bowl along with the ground walnuts, thyme, turmeric, and white pepper. Mix well and spread evenly into the prepared dish. Sprinkle the remaining walnuts over the top and press them in gently.

5. Bake for 25 to 30 minutes or until the pie is firm. Let set for about 5 minutes before cutting.

NOTE: For a change, add ¼ cup chopped fresh dill or ¼ cup chopped fresh parsley to the recipe.

CURRY SPICED PISTACHIO CRUSTED POTATO CAKES

MAKES 9 TO 10 PATTIES
(ABOUT 4 SERVINGS)

These are delicious with a tofu, tempeh, or lentil dish and a salad. Increase the spiciness as you like by adding more cayenne, or reduce the spiciness with less—or remove the spiciness by omitting the cayenne altogether. If the cakes are not all going to be eaten when you make the recipe, wrap the leftovers in waxed paper or in a container with waxed paper between the potato cake layers, and cook them when you are ready to serve them.

2 pounds potatoes, scrubbed and diced

2 teaspoons olive oil

5 cloves minced garlic

1 tablespoon grated ginger

2 teaspoons cumin seeds

2 teaspoons garam masala

2 teaspoons turmeric

Pinch of cayenne, or to taste

½ cup pistachios, coarsely ground

2 tablespoons olive oil, or as needed

1. Cook the potatoes in water to cover until tender. Drain and reserve ¼ cup of the cooking water. Mash the potatoes, adding in the ¼ cup cooking water.

2. While the potatoes are cooking, heat 2 teaspoons oil in a small saucepan. Add the garlic, ginger, and cumin seeds. Cook, stirring often, until the garlic begins to brown, then add the garam masala, turmeric, and cayenne. Stir and cook for a minute or so more.

3. Add the spices to the mashed potatoes and mix well.

4. When the mixture is cool enough to handle, shape it into patties that are approximately 3 inches in diameter.

5. Place the pistachios on a small plate and dip each patty into the nuts to coat on both sides. Set aside.

6. Heat 1 tablespoon olive oil, or more as needed, in a large skillet and place about half the patties in the skillet. Press them down slightly with a spatula to press in the nuts. Cook until each patty is crispy brown on the bottom. Turn them over and cook on the other side. Keep the cooked patties in a warm oven while you cook the rest.

NOTE: I cook potatoes for this sort of recipe in a pressure cooker with only a cup or two of water. They turn out perfect and you are not throwing out the minerals in the cooking water, because there will not be much left. But if you prefer, you can boil them.

EGGPLANT WITH CARAMELIZED ONIONS, WALNUTS, AND PEAS

MAKES 4 TO 6 SERVINGS

For years this was one of my favorite eggplant recipes, but without nuts. One day I decided to add walnuts, and it was fabulous. It is so easy, too! Try this dish over quinoa and serve with a salad for an easy meal. One thing to keep in mind is that because there is not much liquid added to this recipe, you need a good, heavy pan with a well-fitted lid.

2 tablespoons olive oil

2½ cups chopped sweet onions (1 large)

8 cups eggplant, cut into 1½-inch cubes (1½ pounds)

3 tablespoons tamari

2 tablespoons balsamic vinegar

1¼ cups frozen peas

¾ cup chopped walnuts

½ teaspoon white pepper

¼ cup chiffonade of basil

1. Place the olive oil in the bottom of a large, heavy pan. Add the onions and stir.

2. Top the onions with the eggplant, then add the tamari and balsamic vinegar but don't stir. Cover the pan, place it on medium-low heat, and cook without stirring for about

20 minutes, or until the dish begins to give off a delicious fragrance. (Not stirring allows the onions to caramelize.) Keep the lid closed as long as possible, but if you need to check, take the pan off the heat and check the eggplant as quickly as possible. If it appears to be scorching on the bottom, stir and add a tablespoon or two of water, but the longer you can wait the better, and if you get the heat right and don't peek, it will cook nicely without scorching or adding water.

3. When the eggplant is cooked, stir in the peas, walnuts, and pepper. Reheat briefly, if necessary. Garnish with the basil before serving.

NOTE: Try omitting the peas and adding a can of drained garbanzo beans or white beans to this dish and serving it over whole-wheat pasta.

HOLIDAY PECAN TOFU LOAF

MAKES 8 TO 10 SERVINGS

This is a recipe I have done for years, and it is always a hit. It makes a nice presentation when sliced and is delicious when topped with vegan gravy and a side of cranberries. The Walnut Sauce or the Pecan Sage Gravy in the sauces chapter of this book could be served with this loaf. Just double the recipe for the sauce/gravy so you have enough. This holiday loaf is definitely more time-consuming than the other recipes in this book, but it is worth the trouble if you would like a vegan main dish for a holiday meal. Vital wheat gluten is available in health food stores. It can be used to make the traditional Japanese food seitan.

LOAF
2 pounds firm silken tofu

¼ cup tamari

2 teaspoons herbs de Provence

4 to 6 cloves garlic, pressed

½ cup vital wheat gluten

FILLING
2 cups pecans

1 tablespoon olive oil

1 cup chopped onions

1 cup chopped celery

3 slices whole-grain bread, cut into ½-inch cubes (3 cups)

1 cup seasoned vegetable broth

1½ teaspoons powdered egg replacer, equal to one egg

1½ teaspoons dried sage

1. Preheat the oven to 350°F. Generously oil and flour a 12 × 4½ × 3-inch loaf pan and set aside.

2. Blend the tofu in a blender or food processor until smooth and creamy, in two batches if necessary. Transfer the blended tofu to a large mixing bowl. Add the tamari, herbs de Provence, garlic, and gluten. Mix well.

3. Spread three-quarters of the tofu mixture evenly in the prepared loaf pan, reserving the remainder for later use. Use your hands or the back of a spoon dipped in cool water to smooth out the tofu mixture and make sure that it is firmly pressed against the sides of the pan.

4. Bake for 10 minutes. Remove from the oven and set aside while you make the filling.

5. Place the pecans in a shallow baking dish and bake at 350°F for 10 minutes, until they are lightly toasted. Stir them occasionally while they are baking so that they brown evenly.

6. Coarsely grind the toasted nuts in a blender or food processor. Set aside.

7. Heat the oil in a skillet. Add the onions and celery. Sauté until tender. Place the sautéed vegetables in a large bowl with the bread cubes and mix well. Pour the seasoned vegetable broth over the bread mixture. Add the ground pecans, egg replacer, and sage and mix thoroughly.

8. Pack the filling into the center of the tofu-lined pan. Spread the top with the remaining tofu. Press around the edges with the back of a spoon to seal.

9. Bake at 350°F for 50 minutes. When the loaf is done, it should be firm and brown.

10. Let the loaf cool in the pan for at least 15 minutes before unmolding onto a serving platter. Slice and serve.

TIP: This loaf may be prepared a day in advance and refrigerated. Bake for an extra 10 to 15 minutes if it is cold.

NOTE: I have a 12-inch-long loaf pan that I have always used to make this dish and that I thought was necessary. One year when teaching a class, I forgot my pan and had to do it in a round casserole dish, and it worked just fine. So any deep dish container that this will nicely fit into will work; however, if you can find a 12-inch loaf pan, it bakes and slices nicely.

LENTIL PIE

MAKES 8 SERVINGS

This is another good recipe for a winter gathering. It is delicious accompanied with homemade relish or ketchup, or a sauce and holiday fixings, or simply a steamed vegetable and green salad.

1½ cups uncooked lentils, picked over and rinsed

3 cups water

1 tablespoon olive oil

1 stalk celery, chopped

1 medium onion, chopped

1 teaspoon ground thyme

1 teaspoon cinnamon

¼ teaspoon ground cloves

2 tablespoons ground flaxseed

⅓ cup nutritional yeast

1 cup walnuts, coarsely ground

¼ cup tamari

¼ cup tomato paste

Unbaked 9-inch double whole-wheat piecrust

1. Place the lentils in a medium-size pan with the water. Cover, bring to a boil, then reduce the heat and cook for about 40 to 45 minutes, or until the lentils are tender and the water is absorbed. When the lentils are almost done, preheat the oven to 375°F.

2. Heat the oil in a skillet and then add the celery, onion, thyme, cinnamon, and cloves. Sauté for 5 minutes, or until the celery is just barely tender.

4. Add the cooked lentils to the celery-onion mixture and then add the remaining ingredients. Mix well and mash the lentils a little bit with a fork or potato masher.

5. Evenly fill the unbaked pie shell with the mixture. Cover with the top crust. Flute the edges and cut a hole in the top crust to allow steam to escape.

5. Bake on the bottom rack of the oven at 375°F for 40 minutes, or until the crust is golden brown.

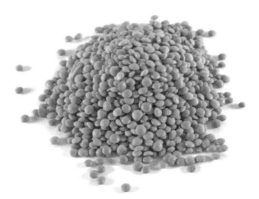

QUINOA-STUFFED ACORN SQUASH WITH PECANS

MAKES 4 GENEROUS SERVINGS

Pecans, shallots, garlic, and sage are a beautiful combo that is great for the holidays or any season. Delicious with green beans or Brussels sprouts and a salad.

2 acorn squash (about 1½ pounds each)

1 tablespoon olive oil

½ cup finely chopped shallots

6 cloves garlic, minced

½ cup chopped pecans

2 cups cooked red or tri-color quinoa

1 teaspoon dried sage

1 tablespoon plus 1 teaspoon tamari

½ teaspoon white pepper

¼ teaspoon salt

1 clove garlic

¼ cup chopped pecans

1. Cut the squash in half lengthwise. Scrape out and discard the seeds. Place the squash on an oiled baking sheet, cut side down, and bake at 350°F for about 30 minutes, or until the flesh can be fairly easily spooned out of the shell, but it is still firm enough to hold its shape.

2. While the squash is baking, heat the olive oil in a skillet and sauté the shallots and garlic over medium heat until they are lightly browned. Add the pecans and sauté for a couple of minutes, or until they smell fragrant. Then add the quinoa, sage, tamari, and white pepper. Stir over medium heat until the mixture is piping hot.

3. Let the squash cool enough to handle. Using a clean dishtowel to hold it firmly, scrape the flesh out into a medium-size mixing bowl, leaving about ¼-inch all around so the squash shells will hold their shape.

4. Add the ¼ teaspoon salt to the mixing bowl with the squash, and press in the remaining clove of garlic. Mash with a fork and mix well.

5. Fill the squash shells with the quinoa mixture, evenly distributing it between the four shells. Top the quinoa mixture with the mashed squash and sprinkle the remaining chopped nuts over the squash.

6. Return the squash to the oven and bake another 15 minutes or so, until heated through and the nuts on top are toasted. Serve immediately.

QUINOA WITH GREEN BEANS AND HAZELNUTS

MAKES 2 TO 3 SERVINGS

Even though this is a quick and easy dish, with garden fresh green beans it is truly superb!

½ cup hazelnuts

1 teaspoon olive oil

1 cup quinoa, rinsed

2 cups water

3 cups green beans, cut in 1-inch pieces

1 tablespoon olive oil

1 cup chopped onions

3 cloves garlic, minced

1 teaspoon tarragon

½ red bell pepper, finely diced

1 tablespoon lemon juice

½ teaspoon salt

2 tablespoons mirin

1 tablespoon tamari

1. Preheat the oven to 350°F.

2. Place the hazelnuts in a small bowl with 1 teaspoon olive oil. Stir to coat the nuts with oil and place them in a small baking dish. Bake for about 10 minutes, or until the nuts are fragrant and roasted, stirring once during the baking. Set aside to cool.

3. Place the quinoa in a medium-size pan with the water, cover, and bring to a boil. Then reduce the heat and simmer for 15 to 20 minutes, or until the water is absorbed.

4. While the quinoa is cooking, steam the green beans for about 10 minutes, or until they are done to your liking.

5. While the beans are cooking, heat 1 table-spoon olive oil in a large skillet. Add the onions, garlic, and tarragon. Sauté over medium heat until the onions are nearly tender and translucent. Add the bell pepper and sauté for 1 to 2 minutes longer.

6. In a small bowl, mix together the lemon, salt, mirin, and tamari. Pour this mixture over the vegetables in the skillet and sauté for 2 to 3 minutes longer. Add the green beans and mix well.

7. Place servings of quinoa, as desired, on individual plates. Spoon the vegetable mixture over the bed of quinoa including any broth remaining in the skillet. Top with the hazel-nuts and serve immediately.

TEMPEH WALNUT SHEPHERD'S PIE

MAKES 8 TO 12 SERVINGS

This is a fairly large recipe that can be easily cut down to half, but it is also a good one to make for a crowd because most everyone likes it and it can be made in advance and baked just before serving. Don't let the long list of ingredients put you off, because this is easy! Serve it with a big simple green salad for a great and easy meal.

3 pounds potatoes, cleaned and diced

1 teaspoon salt, or less to taste

2 tablespoons olive oil

1½ cups chopped onions

16 ounces tempeh (2 8-ounce packages), thinly sliced and cut into small pieces

⅓ cup nutritional yeast

1 cup coarsely ground walnuts

⅓ cup water

2 tablespoons tamari

2 teaspoons dried thyme

2 teaspoons ground sage

1 teaspoon coriander

1 teaspoon white pepper

½ teaspoon cinnamon

1 pound frozen peas

2 cups frozen corn

1 tablespoon olive oil

1 teaspoon smoked paprika

1. Preheat the oven to 350°F. Lightly oil a 3-quart lasagna pan or other rectangular or square baking dish.

2. Cook the potatoes, and mash them with salt, to taste, and enough milk or cooking water to have a consistency you like. Or use 4 to 6 cups leftover mashed potatoes. Set aside.

3. Heat the olive oil in a large skillet. Add the onions and sauté until they start to become translucent. Add the tempeh, stir, cover, and cook, stirring often, over medium heat for about 10 minutes.

4. Add the yeast, walnuts, water, tamari, thyme, sage, coriander, white pepper, and cinnamon. Mix well and cook for a couple of minutes.

5. Transfer the tempeh mixture to the baking dish and spread it out to cover the bottom of the pan in an even thickness.

6. Evenly distribute the peas and corn over the tempeh mixture. They don't have to be thawed. You can use them directly out of the freezer.

7. Spread the mashed potatoes over the peas and carrots, then drizzle the top with the tablespoon of olive oil and sprinkle it with the smoked paprika.

8. Bake for 20 to 30 minutes, then turn the oven to broil for a couple of minutes to brown the top, if necessary, being careful not to burn it. Let it cool for about 5 minutes before serving.

TOFU ALMOND BALLS

MAKES 30 MEATBALLS
(ABOUT 6 SERVINGS)

These faux meatballs have a nice, firm texture and great flavor. Since they do not contain grain, they go beautifully with spaghetti or other pasta when served with your favorite tomato sauce. You need an extra firm tofu for this recipe like the one that is sold under the name "extra-firm high-protein tofu" at Trader Joe's. Make the whole batch and if you can't eat them all within 3 to 4 days, freeze them to use later.

1 cup almonds

¼ cup flaxseeds

16 ounces extra-firm high-protein tofu

⅓ cup nutritional yeast

¼ cup tomato paste

3 tablespoons tamari

1 tablespoon liquid smoke

3 cloves garlic, pressed

2 teaspoons dry basil

1 teaspoon dry oregano

½ teaspoon white pepper

Freshly ground black pepper, to taste

1. Generously oil a baking sheet and preheat the oven to 350°F.

2. Coarsely grind the almonds in a blender. Transfer them to a large mixing bowl.

3. Grind the flaxseeds to a powder and add them to the mixing bowl.

4. Using your hands, crumble the tofu into the mixing bowl, then add the remaining ingredients. Mix well using your hands.

5. Shape the mixture into 30 walnut-size balls, pressing firmly.

6. Place the balls on the baking sheet and bake for 30 minutes, or until the meatballs are firm and brown.

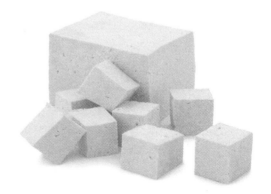

WALNUT-TOPPED BRAISED MUSHROOMS AND MARKET VEGETABLES

MAKES 4 SERVINGS

This ended up being a gourmet dish because I used baby yellow squash, dandelion greens, lion's beard mushrooms, and oyster mushrooms from my local farmers' market. It was fabulous served over imported Italian whole-wheat pasta that was tossed with truffle oil, but it is also great over quinoa, rice, or polenta. I love my cast-iron skillet, but because this dish cooks in wine instead of oil, it is best to use a large stainless steel skillet that has a lid. Please don't worry about the addition of nutritional yeast, because it is delicious in this dish!

½ pound dandelion greens (1½ cups chopped)

½ cup white wine

2 tablespoons tamari, or to taste

1 tablespoon balsamic vinegar or truffle balsamic vinegar

3 to 6 cloves garlic, minced

5 bay leaves

1 pound baby yellow squash, trimmed and sliced lengthwise (about 3½ cups)

1 pound mushrooms, sliced (about 6½ cups)

2 tablespoons chopped fresh rosemary

½ cup nutritional yeast

1 cup walnuts, or as desired

1. Steam the dandelion greens until tender and set aside. While they are steaming, prepare the other ingredients.

2. In a large skillet, combine the wine, tamari, vinegar, garlic, and bay leaves. Add the squash, cover, and cook over medium-high heat for 3 to 4 minutes, or until the squash is just starting to get tender.

3. Add the mushrooms, rosemary, and steamed greens. Sauté, stirring often, for 3 to 4 minutes, until the mushrooms are cooked and the squash is tender but still slightly crisp. The exact time depends on the squash, so look at the vegetables more than your timer.

4. Stir in the nutritional yeast and simmer another minute. Serve immediately over pasta or a cooked grain and top with walnuts.

VARIATION: The farmers' market vegetables make this dish special, but it is also quite delicious with mature squash and ordinary cremini or white button mushrooms, and kale, spinach, or chard substituted for the dandelion greens. If you use spinach, just make sure to press out the excess water before adding it to the dish.

CREATING A
BALANCED VEGAN MEAL

No one is going to enjoy a vegan meal if they feel hungry or unsatisfied afterward. If the meal is bland or the texture is all mush, it will not be well received by anyone but hardcore vegans. Therefore, building a satisfying and balanced vegan meal needs a bit of thought. The easiest way to do this is to think beans, or products made from beans such as tofu, tempeh. Also consider soy milk with grains such as brown rice, millet, quinoa, buckwheat, teff, barley, whole-grain pasta, whole-grain bread, and so on.

Add nuts and seeds for texture, fat, and flavor. Starches like potatoes, sweet potatoes, and other tubers can also work with beans, nuts, and soy foods instead of grain. Seitan is good with potatoes and a nut sauce. Always add lots of fresh vegetables to your meal and a salad, too. Often, I serve the salad right on the plate with the main dish. This may seem a bit gauche if you are used to serving the salad separately, but it looks pretty and tastes good with this type of food.

NUT BUTTERS FOR
VEGGIE BURGERS

Just about any type of nut butter can be used along with grains, beans, and seasoning for making veggie burgers and loaves that will hold together nicely. This can help you to create your own recipes with leftover grains and beans.

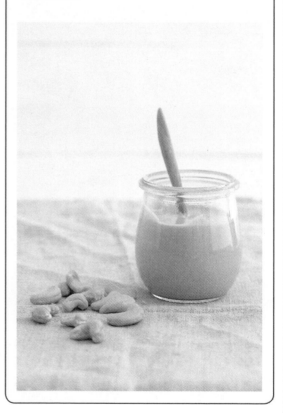

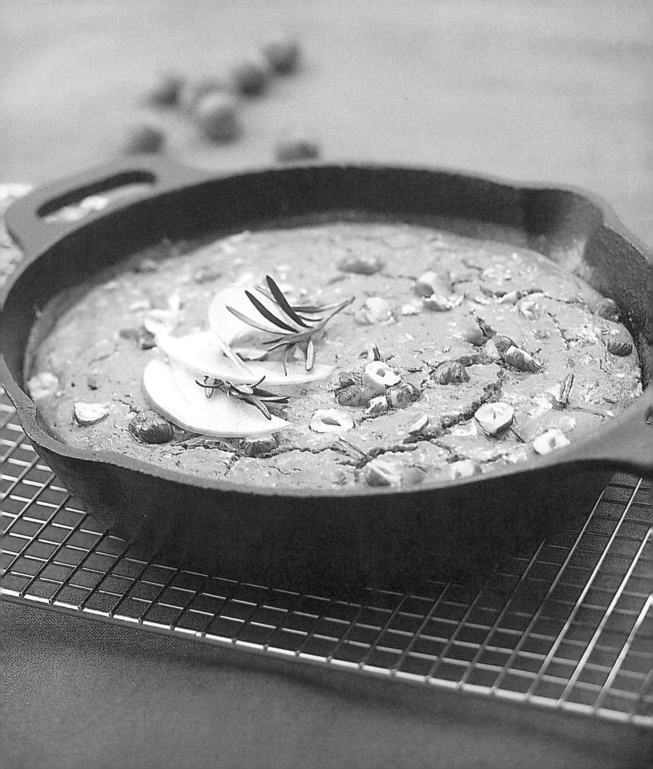

CHAPTER 7

BAKED GOODS

Nuts are a natural addition to quick breads and muffins, but several things make these recipes different from most traditional baked goods containing nuts. First, they are vegan, containing no dairy or eggs. They are made from 100 percent whole grains without the addition of white flour. They are very low in sweetener, often sweetened simply with fruit, and they never use white, refined sugar. Many of these recipes contain no extracted fats, allowing the nuts to provide the fat needed to make the recipe delicious. Therefore, these recipes give plenty of bang for your buck in the nutrition department, providing lots of fiber, vitamins, and minerals.

There are also several recipes in this chapter that are gluten free. The main reason they were created gluten free is because they were delicious that way.

Baking, and eating the results, are among my culinary passions, but I don't consider this a guilty pleasure, because we're talking homemade and healthful. Making sure that the flour is fresh is my first priority in baking, and I can't emphasize this enough. In fact, I have a hunch that if we all ate baked goods made from freshly ground whole grain flour made from grains from the most recent harvest, far fewer people would complain of distress from eating baked goods. Of course, making baked goods that are not overly sweet and/or full of unhealthy fats or preservatives helps a lot, too.

If you have a fear of baking, I hope this chapter can convince you that it is not that hard to do or time-consuming. Of course, the more you do something, the better you get at it; and since you have to start somewhere, it may as well be with these healthful and easy recipes. Learn to bake with wholesome ingredients and you will have a skill you can be proud of!

Among my favorite recipes in this chapter are the crackers. They are no more difficult to make than cookies, and unlike most commercial crackers, they do not contain added fat. The nuts make them crispy. The Hazelnut Rosemary Skillet Bread (page 100) is easy and delicious, too, and the perfect accompaniment to an easy soup and salad meal.

If baking with yeast seems difficult and a bit mysterious, I hope you try the recipes for the Walnut and Shallot Bread (page 99), and the Fruit and Nut Bread (page 98). They are easy and they have a dense texture and great flavor. Also, look for the sidebar with baking tips. I hope you enjoy these recipes. Happy baking!

BANANA DATE NUT BREAD

MAKES 1 LOAF

When there is a stalk of bananas in my garden, there is always a point when they all ripen at once. I usually freeze some and use the rest for a few loaves of banana bread. I took this bread while it was still warm to a small potluck and it was gone in an instant! People have asked for the recipe for years, but this is the first time that I have bothered to measure and write it down.

1½ cups spelt flour

½ cup garbanzo flour

2 teaspoons baking powder

½ teaspoon baking soda

1 cup chopped dates

1 cup chopped pecans

2 cups mashed bananas

2 tablespoons vinegar

½ cup soy milk or other vegan milk

1. Preheat the oven to 350°F. Generously oil and flour a 1½-quart loaf pan.

2. In a large mixing bowl, combine the spelt flour, garbanzo flour, baking powder, and baking soda. Mix well.

3. Add the dates and nuts and mix again.

4. In a blender, combine the bananas, vinegar, and milk. Blend until smooth.

5. Pour the blended mixture into the mixing bowl, while stirring with a folding motion, from bottom to top, using a rubber spatula, and not mixing more than necessary.

6. Turn batter into the prepared loaf pan and place in the oven, on the center rack. Bake for about 40 minutes, or until loaf is firm and a toothpick inserted in the center comes out clean. Let cool for at least 10 minutes before slicing.

NOTE: If you don't eat the entire loaf the first day, slice it and place it in a plastic bag in the freezer. To use, toast for a super delicious treat!

BLUEBERRY WALNUT MUFFINS

MAKES 12 MUFFINS

These muffins have a moist and spongy texture and are chock-full of blueberries and walnuts. They are sweetened just with the fruit and do not contain added fat, except what is needed to oil the pan. If you want a sweeter taste, try adding a dropperful of liquid stevia extract. It is unlikely that anyone will notice the stevia flavor.

1 cup whole-grain spelt flour

½ cup garbanzo flour

1½ teaspoons baking powder

½ teaspoon baking soda

1 cup walnuts

1 cup blueberries

1¼ cups soy milk or other vegan milk

½ cup pitted soft dates, pressed into a cup

1 tablespoon vinegar

1 teaspoon vanilla extract

1. Preheat the oven to 350°F. Oil and flour a 12-cup muffin tin.

2. In a large mixing bowl, combine the spelt flour, garbanzo flour, baking powder, and baking soda. Mix well.

3. Add the nuts and berries and mix again.

4. In a blender, combine the milk, dates, vinegar, and vanilla. Blend until smooth.

5. Add the wet mixture to the dry mixture. Stir to combine the ingredients, without overmixing.

6. Using a ¼-cup measure or scoop to dip out the batter, fill the muffin tin with equal amounts of batter.

7. Bake at 350°F for 18 minutes, or until the muffins are lightly browned and firm to the touch.

NOTE: Vinegar is sometimes added to recipes for baked goods because it causes a chemical reaction with the baking soda and helps the batter rise.

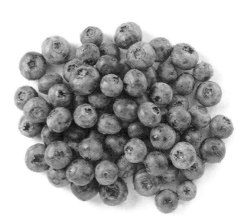

PISTACHIO ORANGE APRICOT SPICE MUFFINS

MAKES 12 MUFFINS

Between the apricots and orange juice, these delicious muffins are sweet enough for me, but if you want something sweeter either serve them with a little jam or add a dropperful of stevia to the recipe. They have a wonderful texture and a slightly exotic flavor.

1½ cups whole-grain spelt flour

½ cup garbanzo flour

1 teaspoon baking soda

1 teaspoon baking powder

2 teaspoons powdered ginger

1 teaspoon cinnamon

½ teaspoon ground cardamom

½ teaspoon ground coriander

2 tablespoons grated orange zest

½ cup pistachios

½ cup dried apricots, cut into raisin-size pieces

¾ cup orange juice

1¼ cups soy milk or other vegan milk

1. Preheat the oven to 350°F. Generously oil and flour a muffin tin, making sure to oil and flour the tops around the cups, because the muffins may rise a little over the top.

ABOUT BREAD

It's all about the freshness! Good healthy bread starts with fresh, high-quality whole grain flour. It doesn't need white flour or complicated ingredients to be good, but the flour should be fresh. I actually have an electric flourmill because I love bread so much that I want the bread I eat to be good for me and those I cook for. An alternative to grinding your own flour is to buy it directly from a small mill and have it shipped to you fresh. See the Resources in the back of this book for providers of freshly milled grains.

Like nuts, whole grain flour contains precious and healthful polyunsaturated oils, which go rancid quite easily. Therefore, always store whole grain flour in the freezer or the refrigerator. To make yeast bread, take out what you need and let it warm to room temperature before making bread.

Starting with fresh flour is the first step to having bread that is as good for you as it tastes, but storing it is equally important. Bread without preservatives begins to mold pretty quickly when it is kept in a plastic bag. So eat your bread the day it is baked, then slice and freeze any leftovers. To serve, toast it.

2. In a mixing bowl, combine the two flours, baking soda, baking powder, and spices. Mix well, then stir in the pistachios and apricots.

3. In a measuring cup or smaller bowl, combine juice and milk. Stir.

4. Add the liquid mixture to the dry mixture and combine the ingredients just enough to make a batter.

5. Using a ¼-cup measure or scoop to dip out the batter, fill the muffin tin with equal amounts of batter. The batter will go almost to the top of the cups. Bake for about 20 minutes, or until the muffins are brown and firm to the touch.

ZUCCHINI WALNUT MUFFINS

MAKES 12 MUFFINS

These are moist without being gooey and have a nice texture and flavor.

1½ cups whole-grain spelt flour

½ cup garbanzo flour

2 teaspoons baking powder

1 teaspoon baking soda

1 teaspoon cinnamon

1 cup chopped walnuts

½ cup raisins

1 cup grated zucchini

½ cup malt syrup

2 tablespoons cider vinegar

1 tablespoon olive oil

1 teaspoon vanilla extract

½ cup unsweetened soy milk or other vegan milk

1. Preheat the oven to 350°F. Generously oil and flour a muffin tin, making sure to oil and flour around the tops of the cups, because the muffins may rise a little over the top.

2. In a large mixing bowl, combine the spelt flour, garbanzo flour, baking powder, baking soda, and cinnamon. Mix well. Add the walnuts and raisins and mix again.

3. In another mixing bowl, combine the zucchini and malt syrup. Add the vinegar, oil, vanilla, and milk. Mix well.

4. Pour the flour mixture into the bowl with the wet ingredients and mix just enough to make a batter.

5. Drop the batter by the ¼ cup into the prepared muffin tins. The batter will go almost to the top of the cups.

6. Bake for 12–14 minutes, or until the muffins are light brown and firm to the touch.

FRUIT AND NUT BREAD

MAKES 1 LOAF (1½-QUART PAN)

This is an easy one-rise yeast bread. It is sweet, dense, and delectable the day it is baked, and just as delicious toasted. Try it toasted for breakfast with fresh fruit and vegan yogurt.

1¼ cups warm water

1 package dry active yeast (¼ ounce)

1 tablespoon coconut oil or olive oil

1 tablespoon coconut sugar

½ teaspoon salt

1 teaspoon ginger

1 teaspoon cardamom

1 teaspoon cinnamon

2⅓ cups whole-wheat flour (approximately)

½ cup chopped walnuts

½ cup raisins

½ cup chopped dried figs

1. In a large mixing bowl, combine the water, yeast, oil, sugar, salt, spices, and about half the flour. Stir to mix.

2. Vigorously beat the flour mixture with a large wooden spoon for 100 strokes. This will help to develop the natural gluten in the wheat.

3. Gradually stir in enough of the remaining flour to make a dough that pulls away from the sides of the bowl and forms a mass.

4. Sprinkle your working surface with flour and turn your dough out onto the floured surface. Sprinkle the top of the dough with flour and knead for at least 5 minutes, kneading in as much flour as it takes for the dough to be smooth, firm, elastic, and not too sticky.

5. Knead the walnuts and fruit into the dough.

6. Shape the dough into a loaf.

7. Generously oil a loaf pan and coat the sides and bottom with rolled oats. Place the loaf in the pan, sprinkle some oats on top of the loaf and lightly cover it with a clean, damp cloth.

8. Let the dough rise in a warm place for about 1 hour, or until it has doubled in bulk.

9. Place the loaf in the oven and turn it to 350°F. Bake for about 40 minutes, or until done. When the bread is done, it will have a brown crust and an irresistible aroma. Let cool for at least 10 minutes before slicing.

WALNUT AND SHALLOT BREAD

MAKES 1 LOAF

This savory bread is dense and flavorful and takes only one rising and minimal kneading. I used heirloom red fife flour, but any whole-wheat bread flour will work. Just make sure that it is fresh.

1¼ cups warm water

1 package dry active yeast

1 tablespoon olive oil

1 teaspoon coconut sugar or other sweetener

1 teaspoon salt

2⅓ cups whole-wheat flour (approximately)

½ cup chopped pecans

⅓ cup dehydrated shallots

1. In a large mixing bowl, combine the water, yeast, oil, sugar, salt, and about half the flour. Stir to mix.

2. Vigorously beat the flour mixture with a large woodem spoon for 100 strokes. This will help to develop the natural gluten in the wheat.

3. Gradually stir in enough of the remaining flour to make a dough that pulls away from the sides of the bowl and forms a cohesive mass.

4. Sprinkle your work surface with flour and turn your dough out onto the floured surface. Sprinkle the top of the dough with flour and knead for at least 5 minutes, kneading in as much flour as it takes for the dough to be smooth, firm, elastic, and not too sticky.

5. Knead the pecans and shallots into the dough.

6. Shape the dough into a loaf.

7. Generously oil a loaf pan and coat the sides and bottom with rolled oats. Place the loaf in the pan, sprinkle some oats on top and lightly cover it with a clean, damp cloth.

8. Let the dough rise in a warm place for about 1 hour, or until it has doubled in bulk.

9. Place the loaf in the oven and turn it to 350°F. Bake for about 40 minutes, or until done. When the bread is done, it will have a brown crust and an irresistible aroma. Let cool for at least 10 minutes before slicing.

TIPS FOR MAKING YEAST BREADS

- Have your ingredients at room temperature; if they are too cold, the bread will take a long time to rise.

- Warm the water on the stove, but don't let it get too hot, or it will kill the yeast. It should feel like the temperature of warm, not hot, bath water, 110°F to 115°F.

- When the dough rises, cover it with a clean, damp towel. I sprinkle the top of the loaf with rolled oats to keep the towel from sticking to the dough.

- Let the dough rise in a warm, not hot place. Here in Florida, I usually put it outside on a hot summer's day, and it is perfect. Heat the oven to low and then turn it off, unless you have a proofing setting. Just keep the towel damp that covers the bread, or it will dry out.

- The quantity of flour in bread recipes is almost always approximate because different batches of flour work differently depending on the humidity. After you bake bread a few times you begin to learn the "feel" of a perfect dough. Eventually, you will make your bread more by touch than by measure.

- To remove the baked loaf from the pan, run a knife around the edges, turn the pan upside down, and tap the edge on a board.

HAZELNUT ROSEMARY SKILLET BREAD

MAKES 8 SERVINGS

This recipe came from trying to create a variant of my Southern cornbread without either corn or wheat so a friend with allergies could enjoy it.

It begins on top of the stove in a cast-iron skillet, and tastes nothing like cornbread, but it has the same thick, crispy bottom crust. It is also quite high in protein because it is made with quinoa and garbanzo flour along with the soy milk and nuts. It makes a tasty meal trifecta served with a soup and salad.

1 cup plus 2 tablespoons quinoa flour

1 cup garbanzo flour

1 teaspoon baking soda

1 teaspoon baking powder

¼ teaspoon salt

3 tablespoons chopped fresh rosemary leaves

½ cup chopped hazelnuts

1½ cups soy milk

2 tablespoons balsamic vinegar

1 tablespoon maple syrup

2 tablespoons olive oil

1. Preheat the oven to 375°F.

2. In a large mixing bowl, combine 1 cup of the quinoa flour, the garbanzo flour, baking soda, baking powder, and salt. Mix well, add the rosemary and hazelnuts, and mix again.

3. In a separate smaller bowl, combine the milk, vinegar, and syrup. Stir.

4. Heat the olive oil in a cast-iron skillet over low heat. Using a brush, spread the oil over the bottom and sides of the pan. Sprinkle the remaining 2 tablespoons quinoa flour over the bottom of the pan.

5. Add the liquid mixture to the flour mixture and stir to make a batter. Then turn the batter out into the heated skillet. Smooth it out with a spatula and cook over low heat for 3 to 5 minutes, or until the edges begin to look cooked.

6. Transfer the skillet to the top rack of the oven. Bake for 12 to 15 minutes, or until the bread is firm to the touch. Slice into wedges and serve hot, bottom side up.

ONION ALMOND THINS

MAKES 36 CRACKERS
(ABOUT 2½ INCHES IN DIAMETER)

You may think homemade crackers are a lot of work, but if you use fresh, high-quality flour and nuts, they are truly superior to anything you can buy. They are no more trouble than making cookies, and these crisp and savory crackers are hard to resist and are super nutritious! Try them with the Faux Chèvre Frais (page 43).

1 cup minced onions

1 cup almonds

¼ cup flaxseeds

1 teaspoon thyme

Pinch of cayenne

¼ cup water

2 tablespoons tamari

1. Preheat the oven to 275°F. Oil and flour two baking sheets.

2. Place the onions in a mixing bowl. Place the almonds and flaxseeds in a blender, and grind to a fine meal.

3. Transfer the ground nut and seed mixture to the mixing bowl with the onions. Add the thyme and cayenne. Mix well.

4. Combine the water and tamari in a small bowl and slowly pour into the mixing bowl while stirring. Mix well to form a dough.

5. Scoop up heaping teaspoons of dough and place them on the cookie sheets in neat little mounds. Using a fork dipped in water, flatten out each mound of dough by pressing the dough with the tines of the fork. Rather than lifting the fork, you will have to slide it off the dough each time you press. Make the crackers as thin as possible.

6. Bake for 30 to 40 minutes, or until the crackers start to brown and are firm enough to flip over. Remove the crackers from the oven and turn each one over, using a spatula. Turn off the oven, and return the crackers for another 30 or 40 minutes, or until they are crisp and brittle. Let cool thoroughly before storing in a plastic bag or an airtight container in the refrigerator.

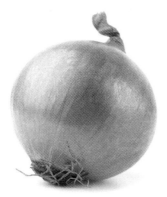

PISTACHIO CURRY CRACKERS

*MAKES 20 CRACKERS
(ABOUT 2½ INCHES IN DIAMETER)*

These little gluten-free crackers are crisp, tender, and full of spice. Use them with a creamy dip or vegan cheese. They would also go beautifully with a salad. If you like a bit of heat, add a three-finger pinch of cayenne.

1 cup pistachios, divided in half
½ cup garbanzo flour
½ cup water
3 to 4 cloves garlic
1 teaspoon turmeric
1 teaspoon garam masala
½ teaspoon salt
Pinch of cayenne, to taste

1. Preheat the oven to 300°F. Oil and flour a baking sheet.

2. Place ½ cup of the pistachios in a blender or food processor, along with the remaining ingredients, and blend until smooth.

3. Add the remaining pistachios and coarsely grind so the crackers will have a bit of texture.

4. Spoon the dough onto the baking sheet by the heaping teaspoon. Using a fork dipped in water, flatten out the crackers as best you can.

5. Bake at 300°F for 15 to 20 minutes. When they are firm enough to turn over, remove them from the oven and flip each cracker over. Return to the oven for another 15 to 20 minutes, or until they are lightly browned and crispy. They will get crisper as they cool. When cool, store in an airtight container in the refrigerator.

WALNUT ROSEMARY CRACKERS

MAKES ABOUT 30 CRACKERS (ABOUT 2½ INCHES IN DIAMETER)

These delicious crackers are great with any dip or pâté, or as an accompaniment to a soup or salad.

1 cup walnuts
¼ cup chopped fresh rosemary
⅓ cup chopped onions
1 cup spelt flour
¼ cup ground flaxseeds
½ cup water

1. Preheat the oven to 300°F. Oil and flour two baking sheets.

2. Place the walnuts, rosemary, and onions in a blender or food processor and grind until mostly smooth. Transfer to a mixing bowl.

3. Stir in the flour and flaxseeds to make a crumbly mixture, then stir in the water. Mix just enough for the dough to hold together.

4. Drop by the heaping spoonful onto the prepared baking sheets. Using a fork dipped in water, flatten each cracker as much as possible.

5. Bake on the center rack of the oven for 15 to 20 minutes. Remove from the oven and, using a spatula, flip over each cracker. Return the baking sheets to the oven for another 15 to 20 minutes, or until the crackers are crisp and will not bend. If there are some crackers that still bend, place them back in the hot oven with it turned off for up to 20 or 30 mintues, or until they are perfectly crisp.

6. Cool completely before storing. Store in a plastic bag or airtight container in the refrigerator.

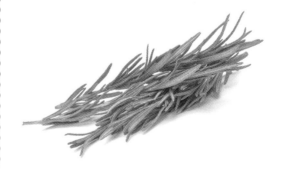

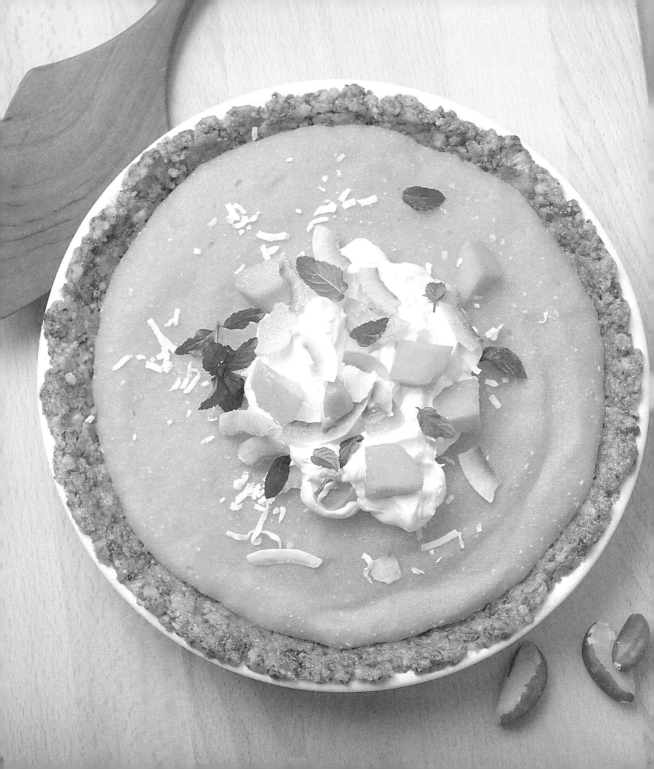

CHAPTER 8

DESSERTS

These dessert recipes are sweet enough to be scrumptious but not nearly as sweet as conventional desserts, which in my opinion are way too sweet to even taste good after the first bite. In fact, when most people taste these recipes, they are surprised that they are so good though not as sweet as they expected. It seems like we often get into a habit of doing something a certain way, like adding a cup of sugar to a recipe, without questioning if it is really necessary or even the best practice. It's just the way it is done, and so it continues for generations. If you bought this book, you are obviously interested in preparing healthy food, so hopefully you will love these recipes as much as I do and be open to a healthier form of delicious desserts!

These recipes are also special because they are vegan and can be enjoyed by people with dairy and egg allergies. They don't contain the high amounts of saturated fats of conventional desserts and they have less extracted oils than conventional desserts because they rely mostly on nuts to provide the fat to make them crisp or provide richness. Nuts lend such marvelous flavor to desserts that it is easy to get by with less sweetener and added fat. The Easy Blueberry Crumble (page 106) is a good example of this because the recipe relies almost entirely on the deliciousness of the berries and nuts to create a wonderful treat that nearly everyone enjoys.

When these dessert recipes use flour, it is whole-grain flour. Over the many years that I have been developing recipes, I have learned that it is not necessary to use white, refined flour to make delicious desserts and baked goods. Whole-grain pastry wheat or spelt flours work beautifully along with some garbanzo flour to create recipes that are not only light, but also high in protein and fiber. All of these, except for the Ginger Walnut Topped Coffee Cake (page 108) are either gluten-free, or have a gluten-free option.

These recipes are also quite easy to make and don't require a lot of special culinary skill or equipment. The Two-Way Three-Ingredient Maple Pecan Cookies recipe (page 111) is a great example of how easy desserts can be. I know how busy I am, and I assume that you are as busy as I am, or busier! So even if you are not an experienced cook, I think you will find these recipes quite doable. But the main thing is to enjoy, because that's what desserts are all about, and delicious does not have to mean unhealthy, as I hope you will discover in this chapter!

CHOCOLATE BRAZIL BALLS

MAKES ABOUT 18 BALLS

Brazil nuts make these treats special. There are similar recipes using cashews, almonds, or peanuts, but try this one and I think you will agree!

1 cup Brazil nuts

1 cup pitted soft Medjool dates

1 teaspoon vanilla extract

¼ cup cocoa powder

⅓ cup finely shredded unsweetened coconut

1. Place the Brazil nuts in a high-powered blender or food processor. Process until they are finely ground.

2. Stir the nuts away from the bottom and sides of the machine and add the dates and vanilla. Process again until the dates are mostly blended and a paste is formed. If the dates are not totally blended, it is okay; just cut up the pieces that didn't get blended.

3. Transfer the mixture to a bowl and knead with your hands until it is well mixed, and then knead in the cocoa powder.

4. Shape the mixture into balls that are somewhat smaller than a walnut. Roll each ball in coconut.

NOTE: The balls can be rolled in any type of ground nut as a replacement for coconut.

EASY BLUEBERRY CRUMBLE

MAKES 6 SERVINGS

To keep the sugar level low, I use both dehydrated cane juice or coconut sugar and stevia in this dessert. The combination of the two makes the stevia practically undetectable. It works with either fresh or frozen blueberries and is a recipe that nearly everybody loves.

1 cup whole-wheat pastry flour or oat flour

1 cup walnuts

¼ cup coconut oil

2 tablespoons dehydrated cane juice or coconut sugar

1 teaspoon vanilla extract

1 teaspoon liquid stevia

4 cups fresh blueberries or frozen berries

1. Preheat the oven to 350°F.

2. Place all the ingredients except for the blueberries in a food processor. Blend until the nuts are ground and the mixture is well combined.

3. Arrange the blueberries on the bottom of an 8 × 8-inch square baking dish. Top with the flour-walnut mixture. Place in the oven.

4. Bake for 30 minutes or until the blueberries are bubbly and the top is lightly browned. Serve warm or chilled.

FRUIT AND NUT SQUARES

MAKES 12 SQUARES

This is a recipe that I make around the holiday season. It is pretty fail-proof, and I have tried it with different types of flour, nuts, and fruits and it always works. Nonetheless, it's probably a good idea to try it as written the first time.

2 cups coarsely chopped pitted dates

1 cup raisins

2 teaspoons vanilla extract

1¼ cups unsweetened fruit juice

2 cups walnuts

1 cup oat flour

*2 tablespoons dehydrated cane juice or
    coconut sugar*

2 teaspoons cinnamon

¼ cup coconut oil

1. Preheat the oven to 350°F. Lightly oil an 8 × 8-inch square baking dish and set aside.

2. Place the dates, raisins, vanilla, and juice in a saucepan and bring to a boil. Reduce the heat to low, cover, and simmer about 5 minutes, or until the liquid is absorbed and the dates have softened to a thick paste. Set aside.

3. Place 1 cup of the walnuts in a blender or food processor and coarsely grind. Coarsely chop the remaining 1 cup walnuts.

4. Place all the nuts in a large mixing bowl. Add the flour, dehydrated cane juice or coconut sugar, and cinnamon. Mix well with a fork, slowly pour in the oil, and stir until it is thoroughly incorporated and resembles coarse crumbs.

5. Place a little more than half the crumbs on the bottom of the prepared baking dish and press down evenly. Spread the date puree evenly on the top. Sprinkle the remaining crumbs over the surface and press them lightly into the puree.

6. Bake for 25 minutes, or until the top is browned and firm to the touch. Remove from the oven and cut into 2-inch squares. Let cool at least 30 minutes before removing the squares from the pan.

GINGER WALNUT TOPPED COFFEE CAKE

MAKES 8 SERVINGS

The idea of coffee cake seems retro to me, but there is nothing retro about this healthy, vegan version. It was created after a friend told me about a coffee cake she had at the restaurant of the National Gallery in London, which I'm sure this is nothing like, but it's delicious nonetheless. It is good at room temperature, best served warm, and is amazing topped with nice cream (see page 117)!

1 or 2 ripe pears, as needed

1 cup chopped walnuts or pecans

¼ cup ginger, peeled and grated

¼ cup maple syrup

1 cup spelt flour

1 cup garbanzo flour

1 teaspoon baking powder

1 teaspoon baking soda

¾ cup soy milk

1 teaspoon vanilla extract

1 tablespoon cider vinegar

1. Preheat the oven to 350°F. Generously oil and flour an 8 × 8-inch square baking dish.

2. In the blender, process the pears to form a puree. If they are organic there is no reason to peel them first, but do core them. Measure out 1 cup. Save any leftovers for another purpose. Set aside.

3. In a small bowl, combine the nuts, ginger, and syrup. Stir, then set aside while you prepare the other ingredients.

4. In a large mixing bowl, combine the spelt flour, garbanzo flour, baking powder, and baking soda. Mix well.

5. In another bowl, stir or whisk together the pear puree, soy milk, vanilla, and vinegar.

6. Stir the liquid mixture into the dry mixture until a batter is formed. Don't overmix. Quickly transfer the batter into the prepared baking dish.

7. Stir the nut mixture and spoon it evenly over the top of the cake. Then drizzle any leftover syrup over that.

8. Bake on the middle rack of the oven for about 30 minutes, or until the cake is firm to the touch.

MACADAMIA CHOCOLATE PUDDING

MAKES 4 TO 6 SERVINGS

This is as good as any chocolate pudding I have ever had and only takes minutes to make. It uses both silken tofu for creaminess and macadamia nuts for richness. With the addition of the macadamia nuts there is no tofu taste whatsoever, but the tofu makes it lighter than the mousse-type desserts that are typically made with nuts only. Serve it in stemmed sorbet glasses or topped with raspberries, strawberries, or pitted cherries. Add fresh fruit to get 6 rather than 4 servings.

12.3-ounce package firm silken tofu

½ cup unsalted macadamia nuts, plus ⅓ cup chopped

¼ cup maple syrup

1 teaspoon vanilla extract

⅓ to ½ cup cocoa powder, to taste

Fruit or fresh mint

1. In a blender, combine the tofu, ½ cup macadamia nuts, syrup, and vanilla. Blend until smooth and creamy, scraping the sides of the machine with a rubber spatula as needed.

2. Transfer to a mixing bowl and whisk in the cocoa powder, adjusting the amount to your taste.

3. Chill or serve immediately, topped with the remaining ⅓ cup chopped macadamia nuts and fruit or fresh mint garnish.

PLANTAIN AND PECAN PIE

MAKES A 9-INCH PIE

In my kitchen a couple of overripe plantains had peels that were turning black and fruit that was getting yucky looking, so they became the basis for this ridiculously easy and healthy pie! When plantains start turning black, you know that they will be sweet and delicious! This pie is great, served warm, with some vegan ice cream. The crust for this pie is super easy to do, but any favorite crust will work.

CRUST

1 cup rolled oats

1 cup pecan halves

1 teaspoon cinnamon

3 tablespoons coconut oil

2 tablespoons water

FILLING

2 large very ripe plantains

1⅓ cups pecans

2 to 3 tablespoons malt syrup or maple syrup

TO MAKE THE CRUST

1. Place the oats in a blender and grind them until they become flour. Transfer to a 9-inch pie pan. Then coarsely grind the pecans and place in the pie pan with the oats. Add the cinnamon and mix well.

2. Stir in the coconut oil until it is distributed evenly throughout the flour mixture and the mixture is crumbly looking, then stir in the water, a little at a time, until the mixture holds together when pressed.

3. Using a fork, and/or your hands, press the mixture evenly over the bottom and sides of the pan, paying attention to pinch together the dough around the top to make a nice edge. Set aside.

TO MAKE THE FILLING

1. In a medium-size bowl, mash the plantain with a fork or potato masher. It doesn't have to be perfectly smooth. Fill the piecrust with the mashed plantain, lightly pressing it into the crust to make it even and firm.

2. Arrange the pecans over the top, lightly pressing them into the mashed plantains, and drizzle the syrup over top.

3. Bake at 350°F for 25 minutes, or until the syrup has caramelized over the pecans and the mashed plantains have puffed up a bit.

Let cool for at least 15 minutes before slicing and serving.

NOTE: If your local supermarket or health food store does not have plantains, you can find them at Latin markets. Just make sure they are very ripe, somewhat soft, and have lots of black on the peel, because they will be too starchy otherwise.

MANGO PIE WITH BRAZIL NUT CRUST

MAKES A 9-INCH PIE

This scrumptious raw icebox pie started out as a mistake, but then I tried it. My friend Emily says it's the best dessert she has ever tasted! You need to have high-quality perfectly ripe and sweet mangoes.

1 cup Brazil nuts
Zest from 1 small lemon
1 cup soft pitted and chopped Medjool dates
2 cups ripe peeled and diced mangoes (2 medium)
1 cup dry unsweetened coconut
Blueberries and mango slices for garnish

1. Place the nuts and lemon zest in a blender and mix well.

2. Add the chopped dates and blend to a sticky consistency.

3. Press the date-nut mixture into a 9-inch pie plate. You don't need to oil it first.

4. Blend together the mangoes and coconut until very smooth.

5. Pour the mango mixture into the piecrust. Freeze the pie for 3 to 4 hours, or until solid. Take it out of the freezer for about an hour before cutting and serving. Garnish with fresh fruit and serve partially frozen.

TWO-WAY THREE-INGREDIENT MAPLE PECAN COOKIES

MAKES ABOUT 16 COOKIES

This easy, three-ingredient cookie started out as a sweet version of a cracker recipe. Halfway through the baking, when I went to turn the nut cookies over, they were so nice and chewy and perfect at that moment. I took some out of the oven, then turned the heat off and let the remainder cool in the oven. This made a crisp cookie. I still don't know which way I like them best, but you can make some crispy and leave some chewy!

1 cup pecans
½ cup garbanzo flour
¼ cup maple syrup

1. Preheat the oven to 300°F. Generously oil and flour a baking sheet.

2. Place the pecans in a blender or food processor and grind them finely. Transfer the ground pecans to a mixing bowl.

3. Stir in the garbanzo flour and mix well. Stir in the syrup to make a thick dough.

4. Drop the dough by the heaping teaspoon onto the prepared baking sheet. Flatten each cookie with the tines of a fork dipped in water. You will have to dip the fork each time you press; and rather than lifting the fork off the cookie, you will need to slide it off.

5. Place the baking sheet on the center rack of the oven and bake for about 18 minutes, or until the cookies are firm and fragrant. If you prefer a crisp cookie, turn off the heat and leave the cookies in the oven until it is almost cool, checking occasionally to make sure the cookies don't burn or get too brown. Either way, let them cool before storing in an airtight container or bag.

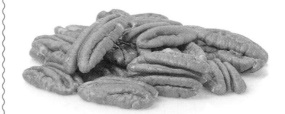

MAPLE WALNUT SHORTBREAD

MAKES 20 1-INCH SQUARES

This is not the pale, bland, silky shortbread we all know. It has more texture, a darker color, and a rich and delicious maple flavor. It is gluten-free and is absolutely delicious with coffee or tea for an afternoon treat. It's also quite easy to make.

2½ cups walnut pieces

¾ cup garbanzo flour

1 teaspoon vanilla extract

⅓ cup maple syrup

20 walnut pieces

1. Preheat the oven to 350°F. Oil and flour an 8 x 8-inch square baking dish.

2. Place the walnut pieces in a blender or food processor and blend until they are finely ground and start to form a paste. Transfer the ground walnuts to a mixing bowl.

3. Add the garbanzo flour and mix well.

4. In a small bowl, add the vanilla to the syrup and stir. Drizzle the syrup mixture into the dry mixture while stirring. Mix enough to combine the ingredients and create a dough that will stick together when pressed.

4. Firmly and evenly press the mixture into an 8 x 8-inch square baking dish, using first your hands and then a fork dipped in water. Cut the dough into 20 pieces. Four slices in one direction and five in the other. Press a walnut piece into the top of each rectangle of dough.

5. Bake on the center rack of the oven for 20 minutes. Recut the shortbread where it was already cut while hot and let it cool in the pan for 10 to 15 minutes before removing.

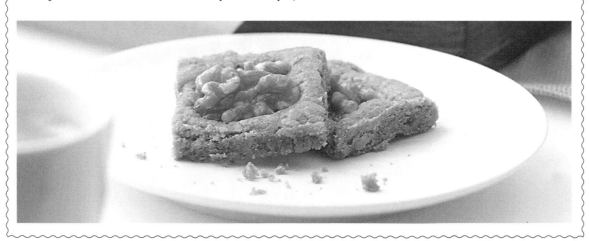

OLD-FASHIONED OATMEAL WALNUT RAISIN COOKIES

MAKES ABOUT 12 COOKIES

Reminiscent of what grandma used to make, but vegan, gluten-free, and without any white anything. These are not as sweet as the traditional cookies, but I think this is a huge improvement.

1½ cups old-fashioned rolled oats

¾ cup garbanzo flour

1 tablespoon ground flaxseeds

1 teaspoon baking powder

½ teaspoon baking soda

¾ cup walnuts

½ cup raisins

⅓ cup coconut sugar

⅓ cup coconut oil

2 teaspoons cider vinegar

1 teaspoon vanilla extract

½ cup soy milk or nut milk

1. Preheat the oven to 350°F. Generously oil and flour a baking sheet.

2. In a large bowl, combine the oats, flour, ground flaxseeds, baking powder, and baking soda, mixing well. Add the walnuts and raisins and mix again.

3. In a smaller bowl, combine the coconut sugar, coconut oil, vinegar, vanilla, and milk. Whisk the ingredients together until they don't separate, then add them to the dry oat mixture. Stir well to make a dough that holds together.

4. Drop the dough by the heaping tablespoon onto the cookie sheet. Use the back of your spoon to flatten the cookies out and press them together around the edges, if needed.

5. Bake for 10 to 12 minutes, or until the cookies are firm and golden brown. Let cool before storing in an airtight container.

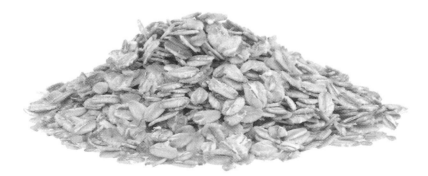

RAW DATE AND NUT SQUARES

MAKES 16 2-INCH SQUARES

This is a perfect, high-energy treat to pack ahead and enjoy after a workout or hike. It uses three types of super nuts and is delicately seasoned. It is sweetened only with dates, so make sure the dates are soft and fresh or it will be too difficult to mix.

¾ cup walnut halves

1 cup pecan halves

½ cup almonds

1 cup soft pitted Medjool dates, tightly packed into the cup

1 teaspoon vanilla extract

½ teaspoon almond extract

½ teaspoon ground cardamom

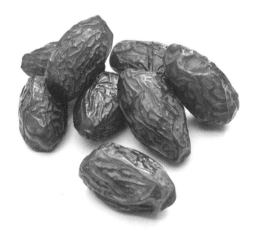

1. Place the walnut halves in a blender and coarsely grind. Reserve about ⅓ cup and transfer the rest of the ground nuts to a mixing bowl.

2. Place the pecan halves in the blender and blend well. They will practically make pecan butter. Transfer them to the mixing bowl with the walnuts.

3. Place the almonds in the blender and grind to a powder. Transfer to the mixing bowl, then add the dates, extracts, and cardamom.

4. Using your hands, knead the mixture together until it is well combined and holds together.

5. Sprinkle half the reserved ground walnuts into an 8 × 8-inch square baking dish. Distribute the date-nut mixture evenly as you press it down. You can use a flat-bottomed glass, a heavy spatula, or anything with a flat bottom that will allow you to firmly and evenly press the mixture into the pan.

6. Sprinkle the remaining ground walnuts over the top and press firmly into the top of the mixture.

7. Cut into 2-inch squares. Store in a bag or in an airtight container in the refrigerator.

WALNUT COOKIES

MAKES 18 COOKIES

These soft, moist gluten-free cookies got rave reviews from everyone who tried them, even the skeptics who thought healthy vegan cookies would taste like cardboard.

1 cup walnut halves

½ cup garbanzo flour

½ teaspoon baking powder

¼ teaspoon baking soda

¼ cup maple syrup

¼ cup soy milk or other vegan milk

2 teaspoons vanilla extract

18 walnut halves

1. Preheat the oven to 350°F. Oil and flour a baking sheet.

2. Place the nuts in a blender or food processor and coarsely grind. Transfer the ground nuts to a large mixing bowl and add the flour, baking powder, and baking soda. Mix well.

3. In a small bowl, combine the syrup, milk, and vanilla.

4. Stir the wet mixture into the dry mixture and combine to make a dough.

5. Drop the dough onto the cookie sheet by the heaping teaspoonful, leaving enough space between the cookies for them to expand, to make 18 cookies. Lightly press a walnut half into the top of each cookie.

6. Bake for about 12 minutes, or until the cookies are lightly browned. Cool on a rack before storing in an airtight container.

NOTE: The amount of liquid in the recipe is just enough for the amount of dry ingredients, so if you add extra liquid, the batter will be too thin. Be careful not to skimp on the flour or overdo the liquid.

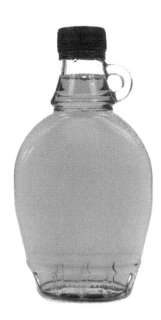

WALNUT BEET PULP BROWNIES

MAKES 16 BROWNIES

Do you juice? If so, here is a great gluten-free brownie that hides a good dose of beet pulp within its dark chocolate deliciousness. It is from my *Pulp Kitchen* cookbook.

½ cup mashed silken tofu (medium firmness)

½ cup beet juice or vegan milk

½ cup maple syrup or coconut syrup

½ cup coconut oil

1 teaspoon vanilla extract

½ cup garbanzo flour

½ cup cocoa powder

1½ teaspoons baking powder

½ cup beet pulp, leftover from juicing (about 1 medium beet)

½ cup vegan chocolate chips

¾ cup chopped walnuts or pecans

1. Preheat the oven to 350°F. Oil and flour an 8 × 8-inch square baking dish.

2. In a medium-size bowl, combine the tofu, beet juice (or other liquid), syrup, oil, and vanilla in a blender and mix until smooth and creamy.

3. In another bowl, sift together the flour, cocoa, and baking powder, mixing well.

Add the pulp, mixing till it is distributed evenly throughout the flour, then stir in the chocolate chips and nuts.

4. Add the wet mixture to the dry mixture. Mix well to combine the ingredients and form a batter.

5. Spread the batter into the prepared baking pan.

6. Bake at 350°F for about 25 minutes, or until firm to the touch. Let cool in the pan before slicing into 16 pieces. Store in an airtight container.

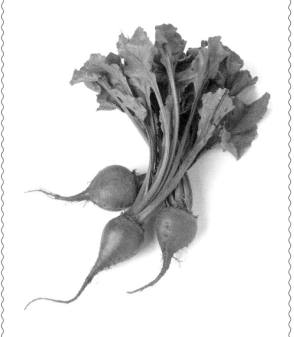

DESSERT TIPS

OAT FLOUR

Make oat flour by grinding rolled oats in a blender, making as much as you need, when you need it.

BLENDING DATES

When using dates in a recipe, if they need to be blended or ground in a blender or food processor, make sure that they are soft. Even in a Vitamix they are sometimes difficult to process, so I make sure they are blended just enough to make a mixture that holds together. They *never* have to be perfectly blended to a paste in order for them to work in these recipes. Also, if your machine is straining, you can use smaller amounts, and/or do most of the blending by cutting the dates with a knife or squishing them through your fingers. I recently discovered this trick: If the dates are soft and fresh, place them in a sealed plastic bag large enough that they are not crowded, and knead them through the bag. This is more pleasant than squishing them through your fingers!

BLENDING NUTS

A small blender can easily grind nuts, but it will have to be done in smaller batches than if a Vitamix or other high-powered blender is used. If you have only a small blender, try blending 1 cup at a time. A food processor can blend larger amounts than a typical blender, but a food processor will not grind a small amount of nuts, because it needs to be full enough for the nuts to reach the blades, or else you will be required to stop the machine every few seconds to scrape the sides.

EASY BANANA PECAN NICE CREAM

"Nice cream" is a name that vegans use for frozen ice cream–like treats. A delicious one can be made in a Champion juicer by using the nut butter blank that comes with the machine and processing pecans and frozen bananas. It is so easy, healthy, and delicious! Make sure the nuts are cold first and start by pushing part of a banana through the hopper; add a small handful of nuts, a little more banana, and so on until you have as much as you want. Adding nuts to banana nice cream makes it so much more delicious than if you use bananas alone!

The same thing can be done in a food processor or high-powered blender, but you will have to scrape the sides of the machine frequently. Try adding other types of frozen fruit to the bananas, such as berries, and remember to serve it immediately, or return it to the freezer until you are ready. But don't keep it in the freezer for more than an hour or so, because it will freeze solid.

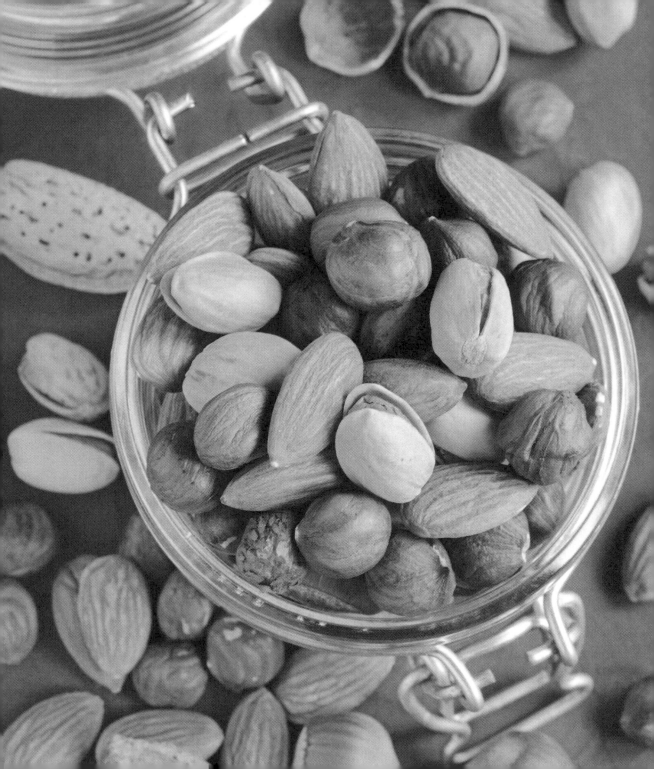

FREQUENTLY ASKED QUESTIONS

What are tree nuts?

The term "tree nuts" has been applied to the group of nuts that, as their name suggests, grow on trees. The term "tree nut" is most commonly used when discussing food allergies since most people who are allergic to one tree nut exhibit allergies or at least symptomology to other nuts in the tree nut category.

Why are nuts susceptible to rancidity?

The fat that makes nuts so good for us is also a very unstable fat and it can easily break down when exposed to air and light. Unsaturated fats are not as chemically stable as saturated fats, so when a food with a high amount of unsaturated fat is exposed to air or light, the bonds in the fat become oxidized, making them taste and often smell bad. Storing nuts in their shells will help prevent oxidation, allowing you to keep nuts for a year or two. Shelled nuts, being more susceptible to rancidity, should be stored in an airtight container in the refrigerator for four or five months or in the freezer for up to a year. Nuts vary in their susceptibility to rancidity with walnuts being the most susceptible, followed by pecans, Brazil nuts, almonds, pistachios, cashews, and hazelnuts.

When are nuts at their freshest?

Most nuts are harvested in the fall so they are at their best for the holiday season. Because of their high oil content, this means that as the season progresses, susceptibility to rancidity grows.

What about the fat in nuts?

Nuts are not low in fat but they are lower in the less healthful saturated fats and higher in the unsaturated fats, which is what makes them a better fat choice. The type of fat found in nuts varies with the type of nut, making some nuts healthier choices than others. While the type of fat varies, the number of calories from fat is based on the total amount of fat, whether the healthful or unhealthful type. Since nuts are a source of fat, the quantity we consume needs to be considered as a part of our overall eating plan.

Does the fiber in nuts change the nutrition content?

Fiber in plant foods helps improve digestion, but in that process fiber can block absorption of some nutrients. Iron and calcium, along with certain fats, might be absorbed at a lower level when consumed as a part of a high-fiber diet. However, the amount impacted or how it changes absorption is not clear for the population as a whole and might be an individual difference. Since fiber is important to overall health, it is wise to not worry about how it impacts digestion and include the recommended 25 grams/day for women under 50 and 38 grams/day for men under age 50, unless you have been told to limit your intake by your physician or registered dietitian.

How can nuts have fewer calories than data show?

Recent research has looked at how nuts are digested and whether the plant components change how nuts and their calories are absorbed. Studies have found that almonds and walnuts do not appear to provide the body the full number of calories that are listed in most reference books. Studies from the US Department of Agriculture have found that almonds and walnuts may in fact provide 20 percent fewer calories than the amount listed in most nutrient databases. Similar studies of pistachios found only a 5 percent difference. Thus far, almonds and walnuts are the only nuts that have been studied by the USDA, so similar effects may be found in other nuts in the future.

Is the omega-3 in walnuts the same as in fish?

There are three different omega-3 fatty acids: EPA and DHA, which are found predominately in fish, and ALA or alpha-linolenic acid, which is found in plant foods such as nuts and seeds. The chemical structure of each omega-3 is slightly different, which is why each has a different name. Omega-3 fatty acids are referred to as essential fatty acids since we cannot make them in our body and must eat them in order to consume enough; however, we can make EPA and DHA so technically it is ALA that is the essential omega-3. Research on the health benefits of EPA and DHA are very clear, with both promoting heart health and DHA aiding brain health. ALA is a bit less clear; research continues to evolve, showing that it may also help with heart health, cognitive health, and a few other areas so that current guidelines suggest consumption of omega-3 from fish and plant sources.

With science constantly changing, how should I think about consuming nuts?

Science is always changing and it will always be changing since research is always building on what we currently know to learn more. For this reason, planning your menu around the current body of evidence is the best way to go. The *Dietary Guidelines for Americans* are released every five years with the most recent edition released in 2015. Nuts are included in the current guidelines both as good sources of protein and for the healthier fats that they contain. In the guidelines it says, "The protein foods group comprises a broad group of foods from both animal and plant sources and includes several subgroups: seafood; meats, poultry, and eggs; and nuts, seeds, and soy products. Legumes (beans and peas) may also be considered part of the protein foods group as well as the vegetable group."

Why aren't peanuts covered in this book?

While peanuts are the most commonly consumed and referred-to nuts, providing close to 70 percent of all nut consumption, technically peanuts are legumes or beans. Peanuts grow underground, not on trees, and they are seeds that develop in a pod that grows from the peanut plant. Since they are not tree nuts, they are not a part of this book.

What does it mean to "activate" nuts?

Activating nuts is a process that goes back to early times when it was felt that rinsing nuts and then drying them made them easier to digest. Scientific evidence has not demonstrated any real benefit to this process but in some areas it has become popular to "activate" nuts. Activating involves rinsing with water, drying or roasting at a lower temperature until dry, and then consuming the nuts. Whether this process reduces the starch content, softens the fiber, or makes nutrients more available is not supported by any research so likely this is just another fad.

Why do walnuts go rancid more quickly than other nuts?

The fat in nuts is predominately unsaturated fats or fats that are not as chemically stable so that when they are exposed to air, light, or heat the fat molecules will break down. As fat molecules break down, the chemical structure of the fat changes and it is this change that makes a fat develop off-flavors or smells, otherwise known as rancidity. Walnuts are the most susceptible to this because they contain more unsaturated fat than other tree nuts, so they must be handled in a way to preserve their quality, flavor, and smell.

How can nuts fit into a calorie-controlled eating plan?

While nuts are calorie rich they do provide a wide variety of nutrients and they contain the important macronutrients, that is: protein, fat, and carbohydrate. Being packed with the macronutrients makes nuts good choices for several food categories; they can serve as a protein option or they can be used as a healthy fat option. When using nuts in place of protein the portion might be larger than a snack, but given the fiber in them they often provide a very filling, healthier fat replacement compared to animal protein choices. The higher unsaturated fat content of nuts makes them good fat choices instead of butter, margarine, cheese, or cream-based salad dressings.

Why are some nuts better choices than others?

The main reason that some nuts are better than others is due to the fatty acid content of the nut. All nuts have a fair amount of fat but some contain more of the healthful, unsaturated fats than others. The higher unsaturated fat content is what makes some nuts better choices. Almonds, hazelnuts, pecans, pistachios, and walnuts have less saturated fat, the less healthful fat, and more unsaturated fat than do Brazil nuts, cashews, and macadamia nuts, making them better choices. The walnut not only has the most polyunsaturated fat of any nut but is the best source of the plant omega-3 fatty acid, making walnuts a very good choice for overall health benefits.

If the calories are the same in an ounce portion, why worry about the fats?

The main worries about the fat in nuts are: Which nut provides more of the healthy fat, and how much can people consume? Even though nuts are high in fat, the healthier fat they contain makes them better choices for snacks instead of chips or candy, as a topping on salads in place of salad dressing, replacement for cheese, or as an accent for meat or fish instead of melted butter. While the fat is healthier, it still is a source of calories, and since fat has 9 calories in every gram, an ounce of nuts can provide between 150 and 200 calories, so nuts do have more calories than some of the things they can replace.

Is it best to choose salted, roasted, or unsalted?

As you might expect, the main difference in two of these types of nuts is the salt or sodium content, but you might be surprised to know that roasted nuts can also be high in salt. Naturally, nuts are low in sodium so they can fit very nicely into a reduced-sodium diet but because nuts don't have as much flavor without the added salt, many food companies salt nuts to make them more palatable. This added salt can be a problem for those who need to consume less sodium due to high blood pressure or other medical conditions. With current dietary guidelines suggesting that a healthy sodium intake is less than 3,000 milligrams of sodium per day, an ounce of nuts can have 70 to 100 milligrams of sodium, making it easy to consume a fair amount of sodium in a portion. Roasted nuts often have seasoning added for the same reason that salted nuts do—to improve the flavor—so this is why they can also be high in sodium.

Why are nuts pasteurized?

Almond pasteurization is required by law in the United States, Canada, and Mexico to keep the almonds free from bacteria that can trigger outbreaks of foodborne illness. The bacteria *Salmonella* grows in the soil, as do many bacteria, but the soil in California, where almonds grow the best, has been found to have enough *Salmonella* present to lead to a low-level risk for contamination of the almonds. To prevent this and major outbreaks of foodborne illness, the California almond industry set out to find a way to preserve the quality and safety of almonds. The industry tested several methods to rid almonds of the foodborne pathogen, ranging from steaming the nuts to pasteurization. The industry determined that pasteurization using propylene oxide (PPO) was the best way to ensure safety of the almonds while preserving the taste and texture of the nut. PPO is a USDA-approved compound that can be used to pasteurize macadamias, sunflower kernels, walnuts, hazelnuts, Brazil nuts, peanuts, cashews, cocoa powder, and some spices, but currently the only nut that must be pasteurized is almonds.

Do all nuts have the same amount of protein?

When comparing nuts ounce to ounce there is a difference in their protein content. Almonds provide the most protein with 6 grams per ounce, pistachios are next, then cashews, followed by walnuts, Brazil nuts, hazelnuts, pecans, and macadamias with only 2.2 grams per ounce. This difference might not be significant if you are just using nuts as a snack, but if you are using them in place of animal protein or if you are a vegetarian, you want to choose the nuts with the best protein so as to meet your daily need more easily.

Are some nuts much higher in certain vitamins and minerals than others?

Varieties of nuts do have different nutrient packages, and while that is good to know the differences probably aren't enough to force you to choose a certain nut over others. Here is an example: Almonds are especially rich in vitamin E, niacin, and calcium, but pistachios have significantly more potassium and they are a good choice for vitamin B6, so trying to decide which one is "best" gets a bit tricky. Since their nutrient packages are so different, you might try using some nuts for snacks, some on salads, some in your smoothie or cereal, and some with your yogurt. Mixing like this makes it easy to boost overall nutrition and provide variety.

Some studies talk about nuts helping to fight inflammation. Is that true, and how does it happen?

Inflammation in the body is associated with an increased risk of disease and it contributes to aging of cells. Why and how it works is beyond the scope of this book, but evidence is beginning to evolve that shows that certain foods help fight inflammation and certain foods seem to trigger it. One food group that has received quite a bit of study is nuts. Studies seem to support the anti-inflammatory benefit of nuts, but exactly how nuts do this is still unclear. Some studies point to the healthier fat content, some studies show that the phytonutrient content is the reason, but other studies seem to support the whole nutrient profile of the nuts. While we wait for studies to show how nuts fight inflammation, enjoy them as a part of your daily calorie intake.

Why do nuts have a health claim?

During the 1990s the International Tree Nut and Dried Fruit Council observed the evolving research on the role of nuts in health promotion and disease prevention. Once the body of evidence was large enough, they submitted it to the US Food and Drug Administration (FDA) to request permission to place a statement on nuts indicating that they can promote health. The FDA ruled that the evidence indicates a possible health benefit from consumption of some nuts, so in 2003 it approved a "qualified health claim." The claim can appear on packages of almonds, hazelnuts, peanuts, pecans, some pine nuts, pistachios, and walnuts. The claim must be stated exactly as outlined in the FDA rule.

Are nuts okay for someone with diverticulosis?

Diverticulosis is a condition that results in small outpouchings in the small intestine. For many years people were told to avoid small foods that could lodge in the outpouchings and cause inflammation, known as diverticulitis. No scientific evidence shows that small particles of nuts and seeds trigger inflammation or diverticulitis of the small intestine. In addition, evidence shows that consuming a high-fiber diet is actually a good way to keep the intestine healthy, hopefully avoiding diverticulitis, but if you have concerns, talk with your physician.

Are nut milks of the same nutritional value as dairy milk?

No, most nut-based milks do not have the same nutritional value as dairy milk and many do not have the same nutritional value as eating the nuts themselves. Nut-based milks are predominately water based and they contain few nutritional benefits unless they have been fortified to provide calcium or other nutrients. While nut-based milks might be an option for those with a soy allergy or for some with lactose intolerance, soy milk is a better overall nutritional option than most nut-based milks.

What about nut butters?

Nut butters can provide a very good nutritional package since they consist of the ground nuts. Nut butters are very calorie dense so it is important to monitor portions, but using them in place of regular butter or jam on toast or in a sandwich will boost nutritional value.

What are the most common nut allergies?

The Food Allergy Research and Education (FARE) organization lists tree nut allergies as one of the most common food allergies in children and adults. Since peanuts are not tree nuts, it is possible to be allergic to peanuts and not be allergic to tree nuts, though between 25 and 40 percent of those with peanut allergies also have tree nut allergies. Those with tree nut allergies need to remember that many times peanuts and tree nuts are processed in the same facility, making cross contact very likely. When it comes to tree nuts, the incidence of allergy to one of the tree nuts varies with no clear evidence that one is more allergenic than another.

How prevalent are nut allergies?

There are eight food groups that cause 90 percent of all food allergies with about nine million adults, or 4 percent of adults, having a food allergy. Children have a higher incidence of food allergies with about 6 million or 8 percent of children having a food allergy. Peanuts cause between 0.6 and 1.3 percent of all food allergy reactions and tree nuts cause between 0.4 and 0.6 percent of all food allergy reactions. As opposed to the other food allergies, peanut and tree nut allergies are often lifelong allergies, though new techniques are working to desensitize people with these allergies.

How are tree nuts indicated on a food label?

The Food Allergen Labeling and Consumer Protection Act (FALCPA) of 2004 requires that the major eight allergens must be declared in simple-to-understand terms on either the ingredient list or in a separate statement that indicates "Contains [*include names of nuts here*]." The statement must list each tree nut by name, not by the broader category "tree nuts."

What is the technique of desensitization?

Food desensitization is a process that is also referred to as oral immunotherapy. During this process, people with food allergies, most commonly to tree nuts, milk, eggs, and peanuts, are gradually exposed to the allergen. Over time people can develop tolerance to the allergen or at least tolerance to a point where if they consume the allergen they do not suffer a life-threatening reaction.

Aren't coconuts a nut?

Coconuts botanically are a fruit, but the FDA recognizes coconuts as tree nuts. Because of this, foods that contain coconut must be labeled to indicate the presence of the coconut. Most people who are allergic to tree nuts can safely consume coconut, but it is always wise to talk with your physician before you try it on your own.

What is cashew workers exploitation?

The process of picking and processing cashews requires muscle, not machinery, and recently a study has looked at exploitation of cashew workers leading to knee, back, and shoulder pain. This problem more commonly occurs in countries where labor laws are lax or nonexistent but the cashews often end up in the United States and Europe. A campaign to support better working conditions is often referenced as the cashew workers exploitation.

Is the iron in nuts absorbable?

The minerals iron and calcium can often be blocked for absorption by the fiber found in plant foods, and this is especially true with a fiber called phytate, which is found in nuts. The fiber of nuts is hard for humans to digest and can block our ability to absorb all the iron in nuts. Since iron absorption is also based on need, you might absorb more if you need more. You can also boost the amount you absorb by consuming nuts with vitamin C–rich foods such as broccoli, green peppers, oranges, or strawberries. A spinach, strawberry, and walnut salad would be enjoyable and helpful.

Why do walnuts carry the American Heart Association (AHA) Heart-Check mark?

The AHA certification is a voluntary program that outlines specific criteria a food must meet to carry this mark. There are seven different categories that a food must meet as well as meeting the FDA requirements for health claims related to heart disease. Walnuts applied for the mark and received it based upon the research that has been done showing how walnuts meet the required categories.

What are drupes?

"Drupe" is the botanical name for a type of fleshy fruit in which the seed is enclosed in a single hard shell that does not split along defined lines. The pit is enclosed in an outer fleshy part that is surrounded by a thin skin. The defining characteristic of a drupe is that the hard pit is derived from the ovary wall of the flower. Almonds and pistachios are examples of drupes.

What is the difference between alpha-tocopherol and gamma-tocopherol?

Vitamin E is actually a name for eight different forms of the vitamin, two of which are gamma-tocopherol and alpha-tocopherol. Alpha-tocopherol is the form most readily used by the body but both forms are abundantly available in plant foods like nuts, seeds, and oils.

Is it best to buy whole nuts or nuts that are chopped?

If you can purchase nuts in their shell they will stay fresh longer, since the shell protects them from air and light. Just remember that cashews are never sold in their shell due to the toxic oil that is under the shell around the nut. Unshelled nuts can keep for a year or longer if you keep them in the refrigerator.

How many pieces are there in one ounce of tree nuts?

Due to the size of nuts, portions vary.

Nut	1 ounce portion
Almonds	23 nuts
Brazil nuts	6 nuts
Cashews	18 nuts
Hazelnuts	21 nuts
Macadamias	10 to 12 nuts
Pecans	About 19 halves
Pine nuts	About 165 nuts
Pistachios	About 49 nuts
Walnuts	14 halves

What is the easiest way to shell walnuts?

Many people prefer buying walnuts shelled, but they do keep better if purchased in their shell. You can crack a walnut shell by placing the nut on its side, the side without the seam facing up. Tap the nut slightly with a small hammer or the handle end of a strong knife. Turn the nut pointy side up and gently tap the point. At this point the seam of the nut should be slightly open, so carefully pull the two sides of the shell apart, exposing the nut. You can now carefully pull the walnut halves out of the shell.

Why are nuts listed as a part of the protein group in MyPlate?

Nuts, along with beans, peas, processed soy products, and seeds all provide plant sources of protein, so they are included in the protein group of the current MyPlate. This inclusion makes it clear for those who prefer a vegetarian way of eating that getting adequate protein is important and that there are a variety of choices to help meet that protein need.

Which phytonutrient is most common in nuts?

Phytic acid is the most common phytonutrient in nuts. Phytic acid is known to help control blood sugar, cholesterol, and triglycerides, making research in these areas of key interest for researchers who study the health benefits of nuts.

GOOD REFERENCES FOR MORE INFORMATION ON NUTS

9 EVIDENCE-BASED HEALTH BENEFITS OF ALMONDS

Authoritynutrition.com

If you are looking for a bullet point approach to almonds and their health benefits, this is your source. Written by a dietitian, this piece gives you all the facts you could need about almonds, their nutrient profile, how they can help with hunger control, and why they can be a part of a healthful eating plan.

Almonds: Health Benefits, Fact, Research

Medicalnewstoday.com

Almonds have garnered quite a bit of interest with regard to how they fit into a healthful eating plan. This article, which is similar to the one listed above, is another easy-to-read, bullet point approach to outlining health benefits of almonds.

"Are Macadamia Nuts Healthy?"

Livestrong.com

Macadamia nuts are limited in their popularity due to cost and availability, but if you enjoy them it is important to know how they might fit into a healthful eating plan. Macadamias do not provide the same healthy fat ratio of some other nuts but they do offer good nutrients and they certainly could be a better snack than other salty, less nutrient-rich foods.

Association between Nut Consumption and Inflammatory Biomarkers

American Journal of Clinical Nutrition, 116; 2016

While journal articles are not typically something I might suggest you read or something you would choose to read, this article does a nice job of explaining why nuts are healthful options, what inflammation does in the body, and why choosing nuts instead of other salty or savory snacks might be good for your health, not just your taste buds.

California Almond Board

Almonds.com

The California Almond Board website offers information for consumers, health professionals, food professionals, almond growers, and processors. The site contains information about the latest research, recipes, and tips for incorporating almonds into your diet along with nice visuals on "what is a portion of almonds."

California Walnuts: Nutrition and Scientific Research

Walnuts.org

California Walnuts provides an excellent, ongoing review of the science of walnuts and their various health benefits. In addition, the website offers recipes for use at home, in schools, or even in professional kitchens. The site also offers tips for storage and information on the walnut industry with information about growers and handlers as well as how the industry views and handles the topic of sustainability.

Chemical-Free Process Approved for Pasteurizing CA Almonds

FoodSafetyNews.com/2015

Almonds are very susceptible to the foodborne bacteria *Salmonella*, and after two different outbreaks in the United States, the USDA mandated pasteurization of almonds to avoid more foodborne illness outbreaks. This article very nicely explains how pasteurization occurs, how the industry has continued to work to improve the process so as to preserve the taste and quality of almonds, and what the industry continues to do to monitor this potential risk. This is an article that can quickly ease any worries about the safety of almonds or the pasteurization process.

History of American Pistachio Growers

AmericanPistachioGrowers.org

Yet another website supported by those in the industry. This site, much like the other nut organization sites, provides information on the nutrition and health benefits of pistachios, recipes to help you incorporate them into your diet more often, as well as information about the history of pistachios.

History of Pecans

Ilovepecans.org

The National Pecan Shellers Association is the trade organization committed to educating culinary and health professionals, food technologists, and the general public about the nutritional benefits, variety of uses, and taste of pecans. The website provides recipes, facts about pecans, information on where pecans grow, how they are harvested, and some fun facts.

In a Nutshell

Eatright.org/resources/food/nutrition

The Academy of Nutrition and Dietetics is the professional organization for registered dietitians, the nutrition experts. On the academy's consumer website you can find lots of quick facts on nutrition, some recipes, and a link to find a registered dietitian. This article on nuts provides fast facts on the health benefits of nuts, information on appropriate portions, and quick facts on the origin of each nut. Great, trusted source.

Impact of Peanuts and Tree Nuts on Body Weight and Healthy Weight Loss in Adults

The Journal of Nutrition, 2007 Nuts and Health Symposium

Who would think that a whole symposium would be conducted on the topic of nuts and health? This article is one of the outcomes of just such a symposium, and while it may not be your first choice for information, it provides a good overview of the science, and offers good support to the healthfulness of nuts and documentation to support the inclusion of nuts in a weight control and/or loss eating plan.

Macadamia

CRFG.org

California Rare Fruit Growers is the largest amateur rare fruit grower's organization in the world. The site focuses on the botanical identification, plant descriptions, and cultivar details of fruits. The site will walk you through all the facts about macadamias, the varieties that exist (there are ten), and also how to effectively grow macadamia nuts. A great resource for the curious or for the individual who wants to try to grow something a little different in their garden.

Macadamia nut nutrition facts

Nutrition-and-you.com

This is a consumer-friendly website that offers information on a variety of nutrition topics. The section on nuts offers some basics related to nuts and nutrition and provides tips for using nuts, helping make them a part of your diet not just an occasional treat. The website offers information on all nuts.

Nutcracker Museum

Nutcrackermuseum.com

If you have wondered about the history of nuts or if you need a new recipe for your favorite nut, you will find it all at this website.

Nuthealth.org

This website is provided by the International Tree Nut Council Nutrition Research and Education Foundation. At this site you will find research on all tree nuts—almonds, Brazil nuts, cashews, hazelnuts, macadamias, pecans, pistachios, and walnuts. You will also find easy access to nutrition research, recipes, and resources that you can use personally or if you need tools to teach others about the health benefits or uses of nuts.

Nuts & Seeds. North American Vegetarian Society

https://navs-online.org/articles/category/healthful-foods/

The North American Vegetarian Society website is a good source for facts on planning a vegetarian diet, recipes, reasons behind a vegetarian lifestyle—the environment and animal welfare are two reasons—and a source for the information on the nutrition and health benefits of consuming nuts and seeds. The North American Vegetarian Society is a nonprofit organization that advocates for healthy, compassionate, and ecological living.

Nutritional Facts of Hazelnuts

Hazelnut.com

Hazelnut Growers of Oregon website. As with other industry sites you will find information about hazelnuts, also referred to as filberts, recipes for their use, and nutrition facts. The site does not have health information on the hazelnut but it does link to sites where you can purchase a variety of hazelnut products.

Qualified Claims about Cardiovascular Disease Risk: Nuts and Heart Disease

Fda.gov/food/ingredientspackaginglabeling

Labeling claims can be confusing but knowing what they mean can make a difference in how you shop for nuts. This piece from the FDA very simply outlines the health claim for nuts and cardiovascular disease, describes which nuts can carry this claim, how the claim must be stated on a food label, and provides information on how the claim on walnuts differs from the claim for other nuts.

Pinenut.com

This is a website dedicated to the facts about pine nuts. While pinenut.com is a commercial site, as opposed to a site supported by a professional or trade organization, it offers diverse information, a long list of resources, and a small list of recipes. They offer a variety of pesto recipes, many of which include pine nuts.

"The Effects of Almond Consumption on Fasting Blood Lipid Levels: A Systematic Review and Meta-Analysis of Randomized Controlled Trials

Journal of Nutritional Science. May 9, 2016

While this is a research article, if you are interested in learning more about nuts and the reduction of risk for heart disease, this very recent study uses the highest level of science to review studies on the topic and provides good support for the benefits of consuming nuts, or more specifically almonds, and the reduction of blood lipid levels.

American Dietetic Association Complete Food and Nutrition Guide, 4th edition.

Duyff, Roberta

This book offers all the information you need to make wise food choices. The book covers topics from nutrition basics to specifics on nutrition throughout the lifespan and for special dietary needs such as food allergies, athletic performance, and many other topics.

The Heath Benefits of . . . Nuts.

Kerry Torrens

Bbcgoodfoodshow.com

This is a very consumer-friendly article on nuts. It quickly outlines the health benefits of nuts and divides them by their fat content so you can see those that are better for you versus those that contain more of the unhealthy saturated fat.

Tree Nut Allergies.

Ari Mayer Mackler

International Tree Nut Council

This PowerPoint presentation is sponsored by the International Tree Nut Council Nutrition Research and Education Foundation, so it can be found at nuthealth.org. This presentation is an easy-to-read, concise explanation of tree nut allergies. It discusses the incidence of tree nut allergies, the science behind the allergies, and information on food allergy labeling. It is a good resource for those with tree nut allergies.

What Are the Health Benefits of Brazil Nuts?

Livestrong.com

Livestrong.com is a website that provides lots of nutrition and health information. Articles are easy to read and generally provide accurate facts. To check the authors' credibility, click on their names. Some articles on nutrition may not be written by nutrition or health professionals, but overall I like the site.

What Do Vitamins and Minerals Do in Our Body?

Vitamins and Their Functions in the Body

Thiamin, B1	Helps the body produce energy from carbohydrates
Riboflavin, B2	Helps produce energy in all cells, changes the amino acid tryptophan in food to niacin, helps with cell growth and antioxidant protection
Niacin	Plays a key role in metabolism, especially cell growth and energy production, helps enzymes function, helps body use sugars and fatty acids
Pyridoxine, B6	Helps body make nonessential amino acids, helps convert tryptophan to niacin and serotonin, helps produce insulin, hemoglobin, and antibodies
Folate, Folic Acid, Folacin	Helps produce DNA and RNA and aids in protection of DNA, works with B12 to form hemoglobin and prevent anemia, helps lower risk of spina bifida, helps control homocysteine levels, which are linked to increased heart disease risk
Vitamin B12	Works with folate to make red blood cells, helps the body use fatty acids, may aid mental function, crucial to cell growth and division
Biotin	Helps produce energy in cells, helps metabolize protein, fats, and carbohydrates
Pantothenic Acid	Helps cells produce energy, helps with nutrient metabolism, helps regulate hormone synthesis

Vitamin C	Helps produce collagen, keeps capillary walls and blood vessels strong, helps body absorb iron and folate, helps keep gums healthy, helps heal cuts and wounds, works as an antioxidant
Choline	Helps with transport of fats, helps to make acetylcholine, provides structure to cell membranes, and appears to help with brain and memory development

Fat-Soluble Vitamins

Vitamin A	Promotes normal vision and helps with night vision, promotes growth and health of cells and tissues, helps with reproduction and development of embryos, protects skin and tissues from infections, helps regulate immune system, works as an antioxidant
Vitamin D	Helps almost every part of the body, promotes absorption of calcium and phosphorous, regulates how much calcium stays in the blood, helps keep bones and teeth strong, helps with cell growth and plays a role in immunity
Vitamin E	Neutralizes free radicals, works as an antioxidant helping prevent oxidation of LDL (bad cholesterol), may help immune function, protects essential fatty acids and vitamin A from breakdown
Vitamin K	Makes the proteins that cause blood to clot, regulates calcium metabolism, helps make some proteins that are important to blood, bone, and kidney health

Minerals

Minerals are inorganic compounds that cannot be destroyed by heat or other food-handling processes. They are divided into two categories to reflect their roles in the body. Major minerals are those that we need in larger amounts and trace minerals are those that are needed in less than 20 milligrams per day.

Major Minerals

Calcium	Helps build bones and teeth and keeps them strong, helps muscles contract and the heart to beat, helps with nerve functions, helps blood clotting, may play a role in blood pressure control
Phosphorous	Helps generate energy in cells, helps regulate energy metabolism in organs, major component of bones and teeth, is part of DNA and RNA
Magnesium	Part of more than 300 enzymes that help regulate body functions, helps maintain cells in nerves and muscles, helps muscles relax, keeps heart rhythm steady, maintains blood pressure, is a part of bones, helps the immune system
Chloride	One of three electrolytes in the body, helps regulate fluid balance, is a part of stomach acid, helps with nerve impulse transmission
Potassium	The second of three electrolytes, helps regulate fluid balance, maintains blood pressure, helps nerve impulse transmission, helps muscles contract, helps reduce the risk of kidney stones and bone loss
Sodium	The third electrolyte, helps regulate fluid balance, helps muscles relax, helps with nerve impulse transmission, helps regulate blood pressure

Trace Minerals

Chromium	Works with insulin to help the body use blood sugar, may help metabolism of major nutrients
Copper	Helps the body make hemoglobin, serves as a part of enzymes, helps with development of connective tissue, helps the body produce energy in cells
Fluoride	Helps harden tooth enamel helping to protect against decay, may help strengthen bones
Iodine	Is a part of thyroid hormones, helps with fetal and infant development
Iron	Essential part of hemoglobin, helps change beta-carotene to vitamin A, helps produce collagen, helps make body proteins, aids brain development and supports the immune system
Manganese	Is part of many enzymes, part of DNA and RNA, helps with bone formation and metabolism of calorie nutrients
Molybdenum	Works with riboflavin to make iron a part of hemoglobin, part of many enzymes
Selenium	Aids cell growth, is an antioxidant protecting cells from damage, helps immune function
Zinc	Helps with cell reproduction, growth, and repair, helps with wound healing, helps the immune system, aids the senses of taste and smell

Phytonutrients

Phytonutrients in nuts are found in three main classes—carotenoids, phenols, and phytosterols. In the carotenoid class you will find these phytonutrients that are more common in nuts: beta-carotene, lutein, and zeaxanthin. In the phenol class the phytonutrients that are more common in nuts include phenolic acid, flavonoids, stilbenes, and proanthocyanidins. Finally, in the phytosterol category the most common phytonutrient is sitosterol.

Specific phytonutrients are listed in the chart below.

Beta-carotene	Acts as an antioxidant, may help slow aging, reduce risk of some cancers, and may improve lung function. Found in many nuts but highest in pistachios.
Lutein	May reduce the risk of heart disease, age-related cataracts and some forms of cancer. As with beta-carotene the nut with the highest amount is pistachios.
Zeaxanthin	Helps with eyesight and may help fight macular degeneration. Low amounts in most nuts and none in Brazils, macadamias, or peanuts.
Phenolic acid	Acts as an antioxidant, an anti-inflammatory compound and may help prevent heart disease. Walnuts have the highest amount, followed by pecans.
Flavonoids	Acts as an anti-inflammatory compound and an antioxidant. May help prevent a variety of diseases. Highest flavonoid content is found in pecans, almonds, pistachios, and hazelnuts. Brazil nuts and macadamia nuts do not contain flavonoids.
Stilbenes (resveratol is the main stilbene in nuts)	Functions as an antioxidant. May help reduce some types of cancer and is found only in peanuts and pistachios.

Proanthocyanidins	May help reduce risk of cancer, improve vascular function, and reduce risk of urinary tract infections. Found in hazelnuts, then pistachios, almonds, walnuts, peanuts, and finally cashews.
Sitosterol	May help lower LDL or bad cholesterol levels. Almonds have the highest amount, followed by Brazil nuts, cashews, hazelnuts, macadamias, pecans, pine nuts, pistachios, and walnuts.

Data obtained from C. Y. Chen and J. Blumberg, "Phytochemical Composition of Nuts," *Asia Pacific Journal of Clinical Nutrition*, 2008: 17 (SI): 329–332. Accessed at https://www.researchgate.net/publication/5556591_Phytochemical_composition_of_nuts

Labeling Claims

The US Food and Drug Administration regulates what claims can be made about foods. There are three categories of claims:

- Nutrient content claims
- Health claims
- Qualified health claims

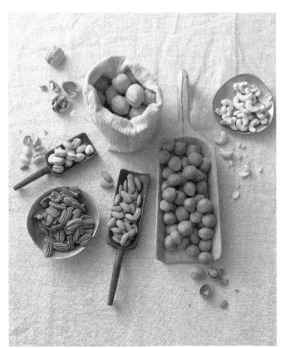

Each category has clear guidelines on what parameters must be met for a claim to be made and each also indicates the exact wording that must be used when making the claim. Nuts could have nutrient content claims or qualified health claims.

The nutrient content claims category has a subcategory that defines terms such as "excellent," "good," "high," "fair," etc. The claims listed here are ones that may appear on or with the sale of nuts.

Nutrient Content Claims

Sodium	"No Salt Added" and "Unsalted" must declare "This Is Not A Sodium Free Food" either adjacent to the claim or on the information panel if food is not "Sodium Free" "Lightly Salted": 50% less sodium than normally added to reference food and if not "Low Sodium," so labeled on information panel

Guidance for Industry: A Food Labeling Guide. http://www.fda.gov/Food/GuidanceRegulation/
GuidanceDocumentsRegulatoryInformation/LabelingNutrition/ucm064911.htm

Relevant Nutrient Content Claims

"High," "Rich in," or "Excellent Source of"	Contains 20% or more of the DV per RACC. May be used on meals or main dishes to indicate that the product contains a food that meets the definition, but may not be used to describe the meal.
"Good Source," "Contains," or "Provides"	10% to 19% of the DV per RACC. These terms may be used on meals or main dishes to indicate that the product contains a food that meets the definition but may not be used to describe the meal.
Claims using the term "antioxidant"	An RDI must be established for each of the nutrients that are the subject of the claim. Each nutrient must have existing scientific evidence of antioxidant activity. The level of each nutrient must be sufficient to meet the definition for "high," "good source," or "more."

Guidance for Industry: A Food Labeling Guide. http://www.fda.gov/Food/GuidanceRegulation/
GuidanceDocumentsRegulatoryInformation/LabelingNutrition/ucm064916.htm

Qualified Health Claims

The FDA has a category for health claims that have some qualifying statements around them so that the claim reflects the science more accurately. Qualified health claims are grounded in science but they might indicate a level of fat that foods cannot exceed, or they might indicate limitations to how a food is prepared for sale; so if it is salted, the claim might not apply, or if the food is seasoned, it might limit a claim.

In the arena of nuts two qualified health claims apply to nuts.

Qualified Claim	Eligible Foods	Label Statement
Nuts and Heart Disease	Whole or chopped nuts listed below that are raw, blanched, roasted, salted, and/or lightly coated and/or flavored; any fat or carbohydrate added in the coating or flavoring must meet the 21 CFR 101.9(f)(1) definition of an insignificant amount. Nut-containing products other than whole or chopped nuts that contain at least 11 g of one or more of the nuts listed below per RACC. Types of nuts eligible for this claim are restricted to almonds, hazelnuts, peanuts, pecans, some pine nuts, pistachio nuts, and walnuts. The type of nuts on which the health claim may be based is restricted to those nuts that were specifically included in the health claim petition but that do not exceed 4g saturated fat per 50g of nuts.	Scientific evidence suggests but does not prove that eating 1.5 ounces per day of most nuts such as [name of specific nut] as part of a diet low in saturated fat and cholesterol may reduce the risk of heart disease. [See nutrition information for fat content.]

Qualified Claim	Eligible Foods	Label Statement
Walnuts and Heart Disease	Whole or chopped walnuts	Supportive but not conclusive research shows that eating 1.5 ounces per day of walnuts, as part of a low-saturated-fat and low-cholesterol diet and not resulting in increased caloric intake, may reduce the risk of coronary heart disease. See nutrition information for fat [and calorie] content.

Guidance for Food Industry: A Food Labeling Guide. http://www.fda.gov/food/guidanceregulation/guidancedocumentsregulatoryinformation/labelingnutrition/ucm064923.htm

2015 Dietary Guidelines for Americans

In 1990 the National Nutrition Monitoring and Related Research Act mandated that every five years the US Departments of Health and Human Services (HHS) and of Agriculture (USDA) publish guidelines for the public on diet and nutrition. The guidelines are to reflect the significant body of scientific evidence related to the components of diet that will keep the population healthy. The guidelines are designed for those over the age of 2 years, though this will change with the 2020 guidelines, which will cover from birth to 2, along with over the age of 2.

As the guidelines have evolved over the years they have shifted from broad recommendations to more specific guidelines on quantity and frequency of consumption of different food groups, and in some years, specific nutrients. The 2015 guidelines took an approach that focused on a combination of a nutrient focus and a diet pattern focus. The main recommendations for the 2015–2020 *Dietary Guidelines for Americans* include the following:

Healthy Eating Pattern

- Consume a variety of colorful vegetables, including beans and peas and starchy vegetables.

- Choose fruits, preferably whole fruits.

- Make at least half your grains whole grains.

- Include fat-free or low-fat dairy foods such as milk, yogurt, cheese, and/or fortified soy beverages.

- Strive to include a variety of protein foods, including seafood, lean meats, and poultry, eggs, beans and peas, nuts, seeds, and soy foods.

- Choose liquid oils instead of solid fats.

Healthy Eating Pattern Limits

- Consume less than 10 percent of calories each day from added sugars.

- Consume less than 10 percent of calories each day from saturated fats.

- Consume less than 2,300 milligrams per day of sodium.

- If alcohol is consumed, it should be in moderation.

The 2015 *Dietary Guidelines* provide examples for how to implement these recommendations in a variety of meal patterns in order to help make the shift to healthier eating easier for Americans. Most Americans do not consume the amount of vegetables or dairy recommended, and the dietary patterns demonstrate how to incorporate these foods easily.

Recognizing the nutritional value of nuts, as well as the role they can play in meeting protein needs for vegetarians and vegans, the 2015 *Dietary Guidelines* included a line on the sample meal patterns that includes nuts. The guidelines include between 2 ounces of nuts per week and a maximum of 5 ounces based on a calorie range from 1,000 to 2,200 calories. https://health.gov/dietaryguidelines/2015/guidelines/executive-summary/

Additional Resources

www.ansonmills.com

Anson Mills sells goods from organic heirloom grains, including rice, wheat, and coarse ground grits.

www.culturesforhealth.com
Cultures for Health has more than 300 products for a healthy lifestyle. Their products include starter cultures cheesemaking and natural fermentation supplies, soy cultures, equpment, books, and more.

www.wholegrainscouncil.org

The Whole Grains Council is a nonprofit consumer advocacy group working to increase consumption of whole grains for better health.

METRIC CONVERSION CHARTS

METRIC EQUIVALENTS—LIQUID

U.S. QUANTITY	METRIC EQUIVALENT	U.S. QUANTITY	METRIC EQUIVALENT
¼ teaspoon	1 ml	⅛ cup	30 ml
½ teaspoon	2.5 ml	¼ cup *(2 fluid ounces)*	60 ml
¾ teaspoon	4 ml	⅓ cup	80 ml
1 teaspoon	5 ml	½ cup *(4 fluid ounces)*	120 ml
1¼ teaspoons	6 ml	⅔ cup	160 ml
1½ teaspoons	7.5 ml	¾ cup *(6 fluid ounces)*	180 ml
1¾ teaspoons	8.5 ml	1 cup *(8 fluid ounces)*	240 ml
2 teaspoons	10 ml	1½ cups *(12 fluid ounces)*	350 ml
1 tablespoon	15 ml	3 cups	700 ml
2 tablespoons	30 ml	4 cups *(1 quart)*	950 ml *(.95 liter)*

METRIC EQUIVALENTS—DRY

INGREDIENT	1 cup	¾ cup	⅔ cup	½ cup	⅓ cup	¼ cup	2 tbsp
All-purpose gluten-free flour	160g	120g	106g	80g	53g	40g	20g
Granulated sugar	200g	150g	130g	100g	65g	50g	25g
Confectioners' sugar	100g	75g	70g	50g	35g	25g	13g
Brown sugar, firmly packed	180g	135g	120g	90g	60g	45g	23g
Cornmeal	160g	120g	100g	80g	50g	40g	20g
Cornstarch	120g	90g	80g	60g	40g	30g	15g
Shortening	190g	140g	125g	95g	65g	48g	24g
Chopped fruits and vegetables	150g	110g	100g	75g	50g	40g	20g
Chopped seeds	150g	110g	100g	75g	50g	40g	20g
Ground seeds	120g	90g	80g	60g	40g	30g	15g

ACKNOWLEDGMENTS

Superfoods Nuts was conceptualized by Laurie Dolphin. Laurie saw the strong interest in nuts—the positive, evolving research on their health benefits—and she decided that consumers would benefit from a book that made the science easy to understand and provided great ways to enjoy nuts. Thank you, Laurie, for your vision, and more importantly, for inviting me to coauthor this book.

Thanks also to Sterling Publishing and Kate Zimmermann for understanding the importance of communicating the science and the need for great recipes.

Sharing the authorship with Chef Vicki Chelf has been a real delight and an enjoyable task. Coauthoring books can sometimes be challenging, but not with Vicki, who developed amazing recipes and who understood the importance of recipes that reflected the science.

Finally, thank you to all the scientists who have studied the health benefits of nuts. Without their work, there would have been nothing to write about.

—**Connie Diekman**

This book was the brainchild of Laurie Dolphin. It was Laurie's idea to put Connie and me together to write a book about using nuts in recipes and the health benefits of doing so. Being a vegan, I was thrilled that the editors, Laurie, and Connie all agreed that the recipes could be plant-based. Making delicious, no-fuss, whole-food recipes with nuts is a pleasure, because nuts make almost anything taste better. So creating recipes for *Superfood Nuts* was fun! Working with Connie was equally a treat because she is so knowledgeable and has a way of making the frequently misunderstood science of nutrition easy to understand and read about. It was refreshing to work with someone who puts science before fad and fashion when it comes to food. So thank you to Laurie and Connie, as well as Kate Zimmerman and all others at Sterling for partnering with me on this delicious project.

—**Vicki Chelf**

CONNIE DIEKMAN

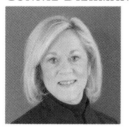

Connie Diekman is a nutrition communications consultant and director of university nutrition at Washington University in St. Louis, Missouri. A former president of the American Dietetic Association, now the Academy of Nutrition and Dietetics, Diekman served on the Academy House of Delegates Leadership Team and the board of directors from 2004–2009. She is a former chair of the American Heart Association–Missouri affiliate.

A former Academy media spokesperson, she has been quoted in thousands of magazines, newspapers, and on the Internet; and has appeared in countless radio and television interviews at the local and national level, including the Oprah and TODAY shows. For seventeen years she was the voice of the "Eating Right" minute on WBBM radio in Chicago. She is a former television nutrition reporter with the St. Louis NBC affiliate and the local FOX affiliate and is the author of *The Everything Mediterranean Diet Book.*

VICKI CHELF

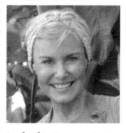

Vicki Chelf has been writing about and teaching others about the benefits of a plant-based diet for over thirty years. She has a degree in holistic nutrition and was the founding owner and manager of a health food store for six years. Vicki is the author of several cookbooks including *Pulp Kitchen*, *Vicki's Vegan Kitchen* (both Square One), and *Cooking with the Right Side of the Brain* (Avery). Her first book, *La Grande Cuisine Vegetarienne*, was published in French and stayed in print for over twenty years.

Vicki is also a fine art painter and graduate of the Ringling School of Art and Design. She lives in Sarasota, Florida, where she enjoys tropical gardening and yoga as she continues to explore the many facets of plant-based cuisine.

INDEX